Dedication

To my girls, Suzanne, Maya and Lena, who keep me looking and feeling young; and to all those, who are keeping it real by promoting and practising skilful human movement everywhere.

THE COMPLETE GUIDE TO

BODYWEIGHT TRAINING

Kesh Patel

BLOOMSBURY

LONDON · NEW DELHI · NEW YORK · SYDNEY

Note
Whilst every effort has been made to ensure that the content of this book is as technically accurate and as sound as possible, neither the author nor the publishers can accept responsibility for any injury or loss sustained as a result of the use of this material.

Published by Bloomsbury Publishing Plc
50 Bedford Square
London WC1B 3DP
www.bloomsbury.com

Bloomsbury is a trademark of Bloomsbury Publishing Plc

First edition 2014
Copyright © 2014 Kesh Patel
ISBN (print): 978 1 4729 0312 9
ISBN (Epub): 978 1 4729 0313 6
ISBN (Epdf): 978 1 4729 0314 3

A CIP catalogue record for this book is available from the British Library.

Acknowledgements
Cover photograph © Shutterstock
Inside photographs © Grant Pritchard with the exception of the following:
pp 12, 18 and 64 © Getty Images; pp 16, 27 and 142 © Shutterstock
Designed by James Watson
Typesetting and page layouts by Susan McIntyre
Commissioned by Charlotte Croft
Edited by Sarah Cole

This book is produced using paper that is made from wood grown in managed, sustainable forests. It is natural, renewable and recyclable. The logging and manufacturing processes conform to the environmental regulations of the country of origin.

Typeset in 10.75 on 14pt Adobe Caslon

Printed and bound in China by Toppan Leefung Printing

10 9 8 7 6 5 4 3 2 1

CONTENTS

ACKNOWLEDGEMENTS

Writing this book was no walk in the park; but the sense of pride, ownership, identity, and sheer relief that I felt upon completion was worth every last ounce of effort that went into it. It's also been a humbling experience by virtue of the fact that so many incredible people had a part to play in the process, to whom I would like to express my deepest and sincerest gratitude.

Firstly, I would like to thank the team at Bloomsbury for their belief in my idea, and for the technical, logistical, and artful direction that goes into publishing a book; to the models, for being so professional and good looking, and to The Gymnastics Factory for allowing me to use their venue as the perfect backdrop for the photo shoot; and to VIVOBAREFOOT for kindly providing the footwear.

I would also like to thank a few exceptional people who exhibit the kind of passion and integrity that others aspire to, who have provided me with physical and mental nourishment, and who have profoundly influenced this book. Firstly, to Simon Rawlings and Tristan Matthiae for being incredible gymnastic coaches and for promoting gymnastics not just to kids, but to adults – you have literally shaped my physical development and your teaching methods are echoed throughout this book; to Steve Harrison and Richard Scrivener for entertaining my rants and ramblings, and allowing me to bounce ideas off them and share their insight – your passion for health and fitness is inspiring; and finally, to the brilliant, maverick and self-actualised Lee Saxby who has taught me the virtues of viewing life through an evolutionary lens – and that there are no mysteries in this world, just a lack of knowledge.

The concepts and methods highlighted in this book have not only arisen from hours of personal practice and exploration, but also from the endless study of methods and techniques from the areas of natural movement, gymnastics, Parkour, dance, mixed martial arts, and other bodyweight disciplines. However, the ability to perform impressive bodyweight skills was never the driving force behind writing this book. Practice and experience has led me to discover that you need to make the right shapes in order to move well. Once you learn to make the right shapes, the fun continues as you heuristically explore the many ways you can sequence these shapes to create movement that is playful yet purposeful, and effortless yet skilful. With that in mind, I'd like to pay my respects to the following people who not only understand the importance of making the right shapes, but consistently put this knowledge into the philosophy, art and practice of bodyweight skills. They have deeply influenced the content in this book and have provided me with motivation to write with humility and respect. To Alvaro Romano, Carl Paoli, David Belle, Dewey Nielson, Frank Forencich, Magnus Scheving, Mike Fitch, Scott Sonnon, Richie Hughes, and anyone who embraces the skill, art and culture of natural movement and bodyweight training in any shape or form. Special recognition also goes out to the late Alfred North Whitehead, Georges Hébert, and Moshe Feldenkrais – your timeless wisdom and desire for the obvious continue to inspire me.

Finally, big love goes out to my girls without whom I'd probably still be writing this book. They have had to put up with my endless squatting, crawling, handstands and cartwheels around the house, and sometimes in public. Such skills may no longer impress you, but I've monkeyed around my whole life. I'm not going to stop now.

Thanks to my wife Suzanne, for being a 24/7 sounding board for the countless thoughts and ideas that helped me sketch out and plan this book – you are my rational filter, providing the necessary perspective that would otherwise not be available through introspection alone. And extra big cuddles to my daughters Maya and Lena, who continue to inspire the old dog to learn new tricks. The love you show for learning new movements and the sense of wonder, curiosity and play that you inject into them is testimony to the fact that bodyweight skill is not an intervention, it's nature's way.

FOREWORD

DEFINITION

Bodyweight The vertical force exerted by a body's mass as a result of gravity

Gravity is fundamental to life on earth. It has shaped our bodies, developed our brains and stimulated the evolution of our unique sensory system – a system designed to inform us about the location, amplitude and effects of gravity acting on our bodies. Science has yet to decide on a definitive label for this sensory system and complex words such as 'proprioception' and 'kinaesthetic awareness' are often used. But to animals, children, athletes and coaches creating movement on planet earth, this sensory system delivers a definitive sensation – one that is vital to the creation of skilful movement and experienced as 'bodyweight'.

The control and application of bodyweight is constantly demonstrated in nature and on the sports field: from the astonishing agility of a squirrel and the rapid acceleration of a cheetah; to the devastating left hook of Mike Tyson and the seemingly effortless 300-yard drive of Tiger Woods – each owe their efficiency and power to the application and control of bodyweight. However, nowhere is the importance of awareness and control of bodyweight illustrated more clearly than when observing a child progress through the 'motor skill milestones' dealing with the associated challenges of learning to crawl, squat, walk, and run.

Furthermore, the influence of gravity and bodyweight is not confined to the locomotor system, but can also be observed in the physiological and pathological mechanisms of the body. The development of bone density, heart disease and obesity are directly linked to how often we support and move our bodyweight – in fact, I would suggest that the cause of all acute and chronic injuries can ultimately be boiled down to inappropriate loading of tissue due to the lack of skill in applying bodyweight (either yours, someone else's or some things!).

I am not alone in my belief that the role of gravity in human health and the role of bodyweight awareness in acquiring human movement skill is not fully appreciated in general fitness, athletic conditioning or physical rehabilitation. However, one person who does fully appreciate all aspects of gravity, bodyweight and all that this expansive subject entails is Kesh Patel. He has seen beyond the shiny, overcomplicated fitness methods and the unnecessary acrobatic prowess that YouTube superheroes aspire to. Instead, he has created *The Complete Guide to Bodyweight Training* as a logical, step-by-step guide to greater health, functionality and performance. Kesh has applied his exceptional thinking brain so that you can switch yours off, engage your movement brain and start reconnecting your body to gravity and the many benefits associated with intelligent bodyweight training.

Lee Saxby

Widely regarded as the world's best barefoot running coach, Lee Saxby has spent over 20 years studying with leading researchers across the fields of biomechanics, sports rehabilitation and evolutionary biology. He understands barefoot movement and natural locomotion better than anyone else, and has used his extensive practical experience to fix injured people and develop performance athletes worldwide.

PREFACE

As I sit here writing this preface, I am a happy, healthy and fit human. I have spent over 20 years of my life helping others achieve optimal fitness and health, and developing and delivering education in this area. During that time, I've also explored many different approaches to physical conditioning, but no one method has intrigued me more than bodyweight training. So much so that at the age of 30 I began a commitment to learn as much about it as possible, a commitment that continues to this day. This book is a culmination of this process to date, and is by no means exhaustive. It's a journey that has included countless hours watching, learning and experimenting with the techniques of somatic education, yoga, gymnastics, dance, climbing, barefoot running, Parkour, Ginastica Naturel, Methode Naturelle, martial arts, Animal Flow, Body Flow, and other bodyweight-based disciplines.

I've always been obsessed with human movement, or more specifically, the process of movement and the way in which it presents itself. Natural movements are effortless yet skilful, purposeful yet playful – and it's these factors that often unconsciously draw us toward such movements with wonder, curiosity, and inspiration. For most adults in today's world, these traits of natural movement are rare though not completely elusive. Consider gymnastics, dance, or martial arts – why are we constantly inspired by those who practise these activities? These disciplines all have one common denominator – their practice is guided almost exclusively by bodyweight skill. The outcome is that these individuals all have a high level of body awareness and impressive power-to-weight ratios. From an aesthetic point of view, such an outcome may translate into natural, fluid movements; from a performance perspective, this can result in biomechanical efficiency, reduced risk of injury, and the difference between winning and losing.

When it comes to optimal health and fitness, bodyweight movements make sense. From a developmental perspective, our bodyweight was the only tool we had to shape movement behaviour during our early years. Key factors in this process were gravity and ground reaction force – and we quickly learned how to work with both by making the right shapes with our body in order to navigate our immediate environment. These shapes invariably allowed us to develop the important skills of stabilisation, manipulation and locomotion that would last well into adult life. When viewed through an evolutionary lens, these skills would likely have played an important role in human adaptation and survival.

Unfortunately as adults, we have either forgotten how to perform these key skills through lack of practice, or we often practise them with poor skill. Therefore, when faced with a situation where these skills are required, we end up making the wrong shapes, and using excessive and often unnecessary muscular force. This leads to poor economy of effort, increased risk of injury, overtraining, stress and poor adaptive capacity. To make things worse, we further exacerbate these unskilled movements through structured repetition and redundant goals, neither of which have any meaning in a developmental or evolutionary context.

While lack of skill, and poor practice, are significant contributors to skill loss, modern living environments are also to blame. Unnatural environments, which are saturated with technological advancements, serve to lessen the feedback we get from our senses, and subsequently create poor movement habits. As modern humans, we are literally running software (behaviour) that is incompatible with our hardware (anatomy and physiology). The solution? We need to update and reboot our operating system by changing our behaviour to run more in line with our developmental (and ancestral) design.

This book proposes that the physical aspect of this software update can be achieved effectively through bodyweight training. By (re)learning and building on stability, manipulative and locomotor skills, we can once again navigate our modern environments with skill and efficiency. This type of fitness is not about humans vs the environment; it's about humans working with the environment. With this in mind, bodyweight training can open up a world of possibility that can not only re-connect us with the basic skills that shaped our early development, but can also enhance our health and fitness by building on these skills, with the aim of improving our adaptive capacity to meet the demands of modern living. In a nutshell, this type of training simply makes sense.

The Complete Guide to Bodyweight Training is not about punishing yourself with mindless exercises, performing meaningless sets and reps, or showing off impressive bodyweight movements. It's about becoming skilful at using your body in a purposeful way. This is achieved using the human motor developmental model as a framework for skill acquisition, and reinforcing this with the principles of biomechanics, the training techniques of gymnastics, and the applications of strength and power training. The drills, progressions and explorations in this book will make bodyweight skills accessible to all fitness levels at any age, and will help to develop higher levels of strength, balance and body control that will be immediately transferable to activities of daily living.

A new breed of fitness is evolving – one that aligns with our evolutionary heritage and early motor development. In a world where humans have readily adapted their environment to suit them, the process of re-learning how to move skilfully with purpose may help us instead to adapt ourselves to suit our environment. Welcome to bodyweight training.

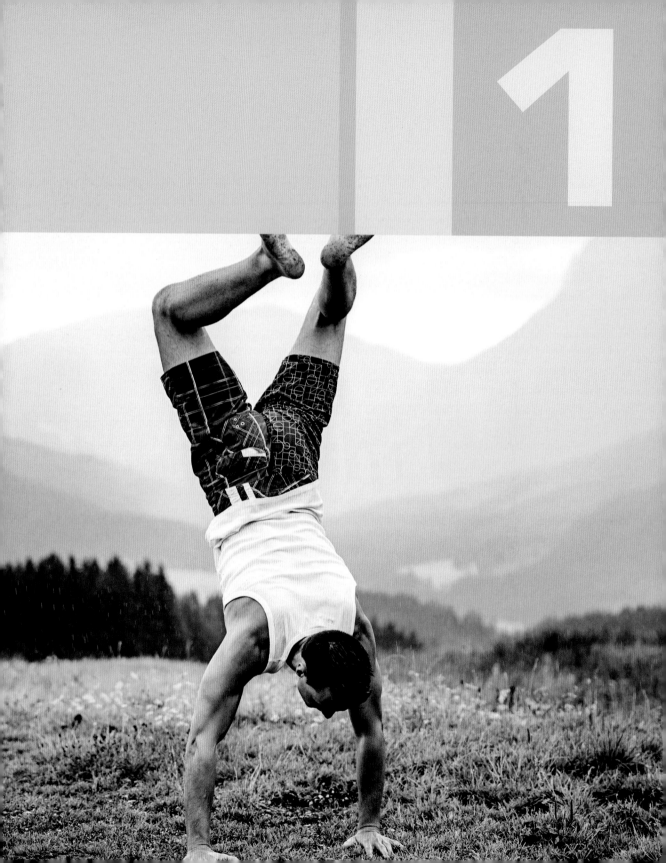

PART **ONE**

INTRODUCTION TO BODYWEIGHT TRAINING

WHY TRAIN WITH BODYWEIGHT?

1

INTRODUCTION

From a human motor development perspective, the efficient manipulation of our own bodyweight played a key role in our physical maturation. During this process, the external forces of gravity and ground reaction, alongside the internal forces of muscle contraction and elasticity, influenced the size, structure and function of our bodies. Through an evolutionary lens, efficient and purposeful manipulation of bodyweight would have been essential for survival.

For modern humans, although the selective pressures are largely redundant, our work and play environments often demand skilful use of bodyweight movement. Unfortunately, the advancement of technology and environmental adaptation has led to a dramatic decline in the skilful use of our bodies, and a subsequent loss of capacity to adapt to the demands of our environment. What was once natural, skilful and purposeful is now unnatural, inefficient, and meaningless. The modern, unnatural environment is literally affecting our health, resulting in a significant lack of ability to skilfully shift and lift our own bodyweight.

With this in mind, the ability to skilfully manipulate our own bodyweight shouldn't really be thought of as a form of training, but instead an essential part of our development and a platform for bringing about purposeful adaptation for optimal health and well-being at any age.

HUMAN DESIGN

It's no coincidence that training solely with bodyweight can improve all biomotor skills. This has resulted in the growth in popularity of bodyweight workouts – replacing many equipment-driven training exercises. Indeed, many disciplines of sport and the performing arts rely on bodyweight resistance as the preferred source of physical conditioning and skill acquisition, e.g. gymnastics, dance, martial arts and running.

We're built for bodyweight movement and exercise – look at our physiology – we have naturally strong feet and ankles, long limbs, mobile hip and shoulder joints, and a unique upright posture that gives us the capacity and flexibility to fully explore our environment. These explorations draw on the simple skills of pushing, pulling, squatting, bending, twisting and balancing our own bodies. And these movements can also be combined and sequenced in various ways to create other natural, yet purposeful movement patterns.

MAKING THE RIGHT SHAPE = SKILFUL MOVEMENT

But in order to move skilfully we first have to learn how. In early childhood, gravity and ground reaction forces were our guides to creating the most appropriate shapes for any given task, from sitting and standing, through to crawling and walking. These lessons in shape development helped to build bodyweight attitude from an early age. As adults, many of us have lost the ability to make the right shape for any given task, much of which is the result of modern living.

Today's technology has significantly reduced the need for us to physically demand much of our bodies – instead of walking, we drive; instead of using the stairs, we take the lift or escalator; instead of playing outside, we play video games indoors. Technology has also led to the development of over-complicated exercise equipment, which has subsequently led to the creation of over-complicated training methods. Therefore, re-educating and further developing our bodyweight attitude as adults would seem the most natural and efficient way of restoring health, function and vitality, while at the same time providing a much-needed buffer to the stresses of modern living.

And why should it stop there? Can we not take these fundamental bodyweight skills and manipulate them further into challenging yet purposeful movements that not only build fitness but transfer to everyday activities too?

USING A MOTOR DEVELOPMENT FRAMEWORK

Motor development refers to the growth and maturation of the muscular, skeletal and nervous systems during infancy and early childhood, and the processes that undermine these changes. The goal of motor development is threefold: to build the strength required to overcome gravity; to learn to balance over our base of support; and to coordinate our limbs during movement. We meet these objectives as children by acquiring the fundamental skills of stability, manipulation and locomotion – which we explore through simple patterns of pushing, pulling, twisting, crawling, sitting, and squatting, before making the transition to standing and upright locomotion. These explorations are often based on trial and error, and for the most part, are uninterrupted by adult intervention.

Unquestionably, these skills helped to shape our early physical growth, but they also continue to be useful well into adulthood. Locomotor patterns such as walking, running and jumping allow us to move from point A to point B as a means of navigating our wider environment; manipulative skills offer a way of operating within our local environment, and include skills such as pushing and pulling; and stability skills provide a means of support and control of the body during both of the above skills.

For our ancestors survival would very likely have depended on a smooth integration of these skills. At times, the demands of living may have required these skills to be used in an intermittent, vigorous manner, for example, climbing or jumping over an object; and at other times, in an endurance capacity, for example, chasing an animal over a long distance. In return for this effort the rewards were likely to be great, e.g. the acquisition of food – and ultimately, survival. However, the modern day landscape is far different. Somewhere along the way we have lost the very skills that make us unique as humans, as well as the capacity to adapt that was once the driver for our early physical development. While our hardware – our anatomy and physiology – is still hunter-gatherer, our software – behaviour – is modern-human. Industrialisation, the advancement of technology, and environmental adaptations are changing the way we use our bodies – we are literally being moulded and shaped in ways that humans are not designed to be.

As modern adults, a reintroduction to progressive bodyweight-based stability, manipulative, and locomotor skills will not only improve fitness and health, it can also make our bodies more resilient, prevent injury, and reboot our software with a much needed upgrade.

BODYWEIGHT CULTURE

Bodyweight training is more than just adding a few push-ups and pull-ups to your training programme. It requires a healthy appreciation and understanding of the laws of nature and physics; and in return, you'll build impressive yet purposeful levels of stability, strength and coordination.

In the past decade, the growing understanding of biomechanical principles has meant that bodyweight training has acquired cult status in certain fitness circles. What was once the domain of gymnastics has now spread to mainstream fitness, with an abundance of websites and YouTube tutorials dedicated to learning bodyweight skills.

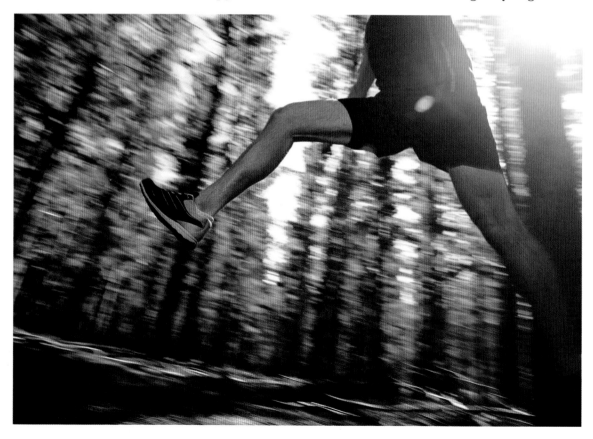

In addition, the former meccas of bodyweight training – the beaches and parks – are now being revived as popular social hubs for such activities. In response to this demand, we are seeing more and more outdoor training set-ups conducive to bodyweight training being installed across the nation.

What's interesting to note is that in the main these bodyweight advocates are not interested in performing sets and repetitions. It's not about how much you can lift, or how good you look. A new definition of 'body-beautiful' has emerged – one that centres around skilful body manipulation and movement flow. It's this very aspect of bodyweight training that is appealing to many, and is exemplified in the art of gymnastics, dance, circus, martial arts, and Parkour – all of which have been strong drivers in the creation of bodyweight culture and its cross-over to mainstream fitness.

BENEFITS OF BODYWEIGHT TRAINING

Bodyweight training can enhance physical and physiological fitness, and mental health in any age group, as well as offer a lot of benefits that other forms of resistance training can't. Specific benefits of bodyweight training include the following:

- Allows for quick, efficient workouts because there is no/little need for equipment
- Uses multiple biomotor abilities, e.g. strength, endurance, power, agility, flexibility, etc.
- Allows for more variation in movement than sometimes restrictive equipment based workouts
- Enhances stability and balance in a natural way
- Is fun and cheap
- Enhances proprioception and position-sense
- Provides a foundation for skill transfer to other activities
- Triggers fast twitch fibres for poise, power and quickness.

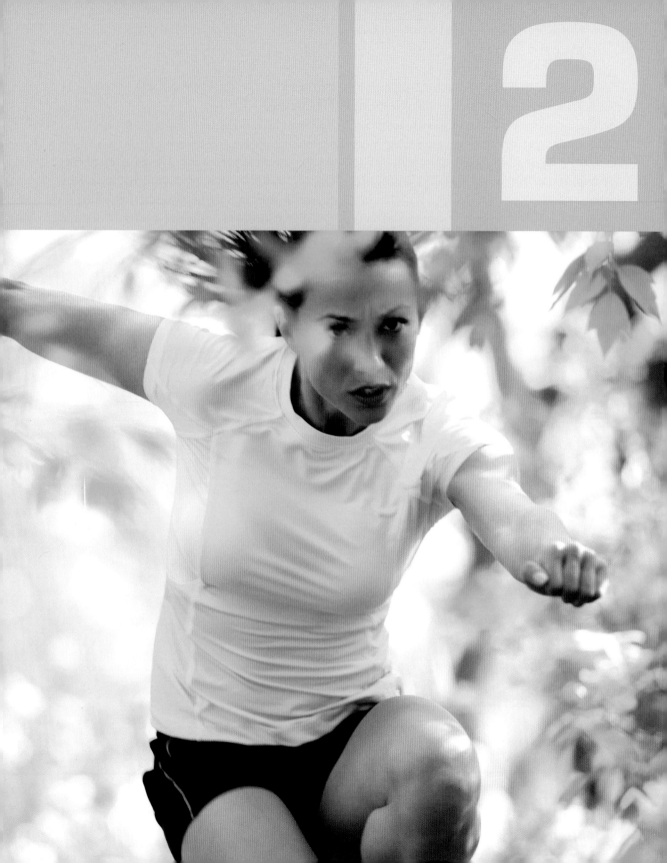

PART **TWO**

EXERCISE CONSIDERATIONS AND PROGRAMME DESIGN

TRAINING
STRATEGIES

The fitness industry is not short on anecdotes and opinions on how to train for fitness, from information on sets and repetitions through to exercise choice and load selection. However, from an evolutionary and motor development perspective, such exercise variables have no meaning. Whether you're a modern day hunter-gatherer, a baby, or an office worker, your survival (fitness) depends on your *adaptive capacity* and your ability to complete tasks in a skilful manner. In this context, repetitions become redundant and have little meaning unless they relate to the successful completion of a task.

When we think of fitness in terms of adaptive capacity, we are forced to explore factors that go beyond the notion of just performing sets and reps at given loads. While such variables can help to provide some structure to training, they often detract from the acquisition of movement skill. This is especially true when learning bodyweight skills, where factors such as mental preparation, movement strategy, body shape, and environmental awareness strongly influence skill development.

With this in mind, the focus of this chapter is to explore some of these influences, and how they can be applied within the context of bodyweight training.

Definition

Adaptive capacity is the capacity of the body to adapt in an environment that is changing, and as a result, to further develop or enhance the ability, capability or fitness to carry out a given task.

PHYSICAL AND MENTAL PREPARATION

As human beings, our sense of fear (and pain) instinctively protects us from harm, and can often prevent us from taking risks. Many of us have experienced trying to complete a complex movement (e.g. a handstand) only to freeze up, bail out, or even desperately force our way through the movement. Were we not strong enough or skilful enough? Possibly. Were we unprepared? Most likely. In all honesty, inverting your body into a handstand is no mean feat, and is a huge risk to take. Our instincts for self-preservation will kick in, and we will naturally ask ourselves several common questions such as: What happens if I fail? At which point is it safe to bail out? What is the best way to bail out?

The solution is to be more prepared – both physically and mentally. Physical preparation involves being competent at each progression towards the skill in question – for example, knowing that you can hold the most appropriate body shape when kicking up to handstand will give you the confidence to perform the skill. Mental preparation means having at least one exit strategy, in the case of a handstand the ability to step or roll out. If you haven't yet mastered this, then your improvement will always be limited.

While a workout partner or other form of spotting technique may help, they may not help to overcome your instinct when you feel yourself losing balance at the top of a free-standing handstand. Therefore, it's important to regularly drill exercises that are part of an exit strategy for a specific skill. So, if you're learning how to handstand, learn how to roll/step out; if you're learning how to jump, learn how to land safely. To this end, the importance of mastering the stability exercises in this book cannot be overstated (see pages 67–96). These exercises focus on learning specific body shapes that will help you execute and exit any movement safely.

The more exit strategies you have (and have practised with confidence) the more you'll overcome your protective instincts, and soon enough, you'll begin asking the question: what will I do next if I succeed?

COMFORT ZONES

A comfort zone is a psychological safety net within which an individual can deliver a steady level of performance (often with a limited set of behaviours) without excessive stress or anxiety. Comfort zones are a type of *mental* conditioning – they can often prevent individuals from attempting

to, or wanting to step outside of them – because it's easier to operate within these boundaries (the safe path of least resistance). For example, continuing to handstand against a wall because it's easier than learning to perform a free-standing one. What's often forgotten is the importance of *physical* conditioning too, especially when learning a new skill. Using the same example, knowing that you can hold the correct shape during a handstand, as well as being able to roll/step out safely, will go a long way in helping you to step out of your comfort zone – in this case, progressing to a free handstand.

With its high level of scalability and diversity of movement, bodyweight training offers a unique opportunity to challenge your comfort zones. In addition, investing time in bodyweight skills requires a heightened sense of awareness, deliberation, concentration and effort – all of which are conducive to crossing the boundaries of your comfort zone safely and with confidence. As you work on the progressions in this book, start to step outside of your comfort zone periodically. Experience the new feelings and responses that come with learning a new skill, and use this to create a wider, more flexible comfort zone.

DRILLING BODY SHAPES

Attaining the right body shape is an essential component of skilful (and natural) movement. Skilful movement is efficient, has economy of effort, and is aesthetically appealing. In bodyweight training, stability training provides the foundation for skilful movement by drilling key body shapes. This begins with the use of isometric exercises (static holds in support positions) that help muscles to engage and hold a specific body shape. As this improves, movement can be added to challenge shape endurance – which is an important prerequisite to efficient movement skill.

For example, the hollow body shape (or dish) is not only an important shape for the efficiency of individual pushing and pulling exercises, it's also an essential shape to create and maintain during the transition phase of many complex movements,

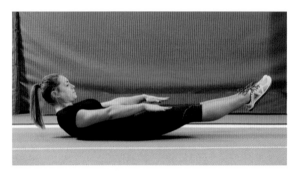

Figure 2.1 Hollow body shape

Benefits of learning how to statically support the body

Static supports are exercises that require the body to be held in various body positions (shapes) from several seconds to up to a minute. They meet several objectives within a bodyweight training programme:

- Can be used within the muscle-activation phase of a warm-up
- Build a foundation for functional strength
- Help to groove correct body tension, position, posture and balance
- Increase muscular endurance and joint stability
- Increase efficiency of force transfer between the upper and lower body during dynamic bodyweight skills.

e.g. candlestick, cartwheel, muscle-up. With this in mind, ensure that you spend plenty of time drilling basic shapes, either as part of your warm-up, in between exercises in a bodyweight session or as a standalone workout.

DYNAMIC MOBILISATION

Bodyweight training exercises such as pull-ups, handstands and cartwheels, will often demand full ranges of motion, as well as static and dynamic control of these ranges. While these demands can be met through regular and progressive bodyweight conditioning, they can also take their toll on the body if left unchecked, potentially leading to joint stiffness, muscle soreness, movement impairment and increased risk of injury. Commonly affected sites include the ankles, hips, shoulders and wrists. A simple solution is to incorporate regular mobilisation sessions into your weekly training schedule.

Although mobilisation techniques should be included as part of any warm-up, performing these exercises as a standalone workout can help to maintain and improve joint and soft tissue health, develop flexibility, as well as groove important muscle-activation patterns required for many bodyweight skills. In addition, because these exercises are generally performed at a lower level of intensity, they can be used on active rest days to support recovery between intensive training sessions. A sample dynamic mobilisation workout can be found in the appendix.

UNILATERAL MOVEMENT

Almost every daily activity or sport involves sequences of unilateral movements – those that involve one side of the body at a time – for example, walking and running, kicking/striking, or picking up a bag. Common equipment based workouts will often involve bilateral movements – those that involve both sides of the body at the same time. If we bias training towards bilateral movements, we miss the opportunity to drill important unilateral movements, and may even increase the risk of movement impairment and injury.

Bodyweight training not only has many unilateral exercises, but also has the flexibility to modify many of its bilateral movements into unilateral progressions. Many stability drills (e.g. front support) can be modified to include a weight shift or a complete removal of a point of contact, e.g. single arm/leg front support. In many cases, these shifts in weight will form the first part of the switch into another position, which is an important aspect when training transitional and locomotor sequences. Removing a point of contact not only adds an element of rotation and balance, it also requires coordinated muscle action to control these factors.

When learning more complex unilateral patterns such as shoulder rolls or cartwheels, it's important to practise the movements on both sides of the body, not just your preferred side. This will not only provide an additional challenge for your workout, it will also provide more exit options and reduce your risk of overuse injury.

SKILL TRANSFER
Traditional fitness training often focuses on completing a given number of sets and repetitions; however, we've previously discussed that nature doesn't care for such numbers. When you next perform push-ups or pull-ups, ask yourself why you are working through these sets and reps.

If you are trying to develop skill in your push-up, focus on making the right shape and on the quality of movement – for example, are you in a balanced position throughout the movement? Do you have proper alignment of your body segments? Are you working through a full range of motion? Perform as many as you can while focusing on these factors. In addition, look for ways to progress your push-up. If you're drilling push-ups to improve your burpee skill, then there's little point in performing mindless repetitions of push-ups. Instead, focus on modifying the push-up – learn to change your shape during the transition to create the required drive back to standing. This ability to manage and change orientations quickly is an important skill to have for skill transfer to other bodyweight movements.

Your push-up may not feel like it's getting easier any time soon, but you'll definitely notice the difference when you work on the next progression. When you train in this way, you'll always be chasing quality and looking for the best shapes and cleanest form – which will help you progress quickly to the next level.

GENERATING MOMENTUM
Momentum is an important aspect of bodyweight training, especially in relation to locomotor patterns and movement sequences. Momentum can be thought of as the force of movement, or 'weight in motion', and as you may remember from physics lessons at school, is equal to mass multiplied by velocity. When executing a sequence of movements, you need to build up your speed in order to get enough power to efficiently move through the transition and complete the move.

However, when drilling individual bodyweight movements that start from a position of rest, how can we effectively generate momentum that will allow us to efficiently transfer into the next position or movement? Let's look at a basic cartwheel. It's easy to see how the forward lunge with long arm reach generates forward momentum that helps to drive the legs over the head. However, by falling into the cartwheel from a standing position (by leaning forwards at the ankle and then stepping/reaching), we can increase the speed into the movement and generate more forward momentum, which can help to drive consecutive movements and potentially reduce muscle effort.

This principle may also be applied to simple pushing movements such as the burpee or handstand push-up. At the bottom of the push-up in the burpee we can generate more upward momentum by quickly straightening the arms and lifting the chest (which arches the back), then using the pre-stretch in the abdominals to rapidly drive the hips up – this will produce a faster return to the squat position. In the handstand push-up, a slight backwards fall at the bottom of the movement quickly followed by arm/shoulder extension, will generate more momentum and a more efficient return to top position.

When performing simple or more complex bodyweight movements, not only is it important to generate momentum, but also to conserve it during the transition to other movements. This is primarily achieved through the maintenance of the correct and tight body shape, and further highlights the importance of drilling these exercises early on in a bodyweight training programme.

GREASING THE GROOVE

Greasing the groove (also known as synaptic facilitation) is a bodyweight training tool that provides a means by which to improve your

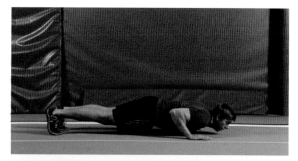

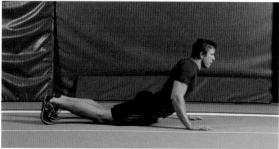

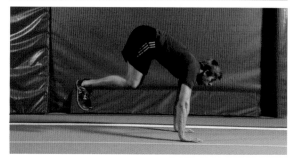

Figure 2.2 Generating momentum in the burpee

movement skill spread over smaller, but frequent chunks, rather than in one large one. It is a technique pioneered by renowned Russian strength and conditioning coach Pavel Tsatsouline. The technique focuses on combining specificity of movement with repetition and works well when applied to bodyweight skills.

For example, if you want to improve your pull-up technique, then you would need to frequently practise pull-ups to get better at them. The method involves training the pull-up as frequently as possible but not to failure (so usually around 50–80% of your maximum intensity). This allows your nervous system to become more proficient at the movement in a relatively short period of time. Because bodyweight exercises require no or minimal equipment, it's easier to fit in performing them at high frequency during the day. The key is to perform a lot of work with a reasonably heavy load.

Use greasing the groove to drill specific exercise progressions that make up a skill, or simply use it to become more proficient more quickly at a particular complex skill.

OVER-REACHING AND OVERTRAINING

Any form of regular intensive exercise can make individuals vulnerable to physical overload, resulting in over-reaching and overtraining.

Over-reaching is an accumulation of training stress that results in a short-term decrease in capacity. It is commonly caused by doing too much too soon, combining multiple skill work in one training session, or even training while under psychological, emotional or nutritional stress. However, motivation to exercise will generally remain high, and with adequate rest, restoration of capacity takes several days.

Overtraining can be thought of as an accumulation of training stress that results in a long-term decrease in capacity, and is usually a product of continual over-reaching without adequate rest and recovery. Symptoms may include loss of motivation and enthusiasm, constant fatigue and poor sleep patterns. Restoration may take several weeks to several months.

It's important to understand that over-reaching is not a bad thing; it's what's needed to force an adaptive response in the body. What's more important is to pay attention to your body once you've over-reached. Continued over-reaching will lead to overtraining, from which it takes longer to recover.

In the context of bodyweight training, over-reaching should be carefully managed. Learning new and often complex bodyweight skills will require periods of over-reaching where you may have to physically push yourself beyond current capacity. If this is done in measured doses (i.e. short, mindful bouts of movement with adequate rest and recovery and sensible nutrition) then over-reaching will produce the required adaptive responses without the symptoms of overtraining.

ENVIRONMENTAL CONSIDERATIONS

Whether bodyweight training is performed indoors or outdoors, it will demand a heightened sense of awareness of your internal and external environment. You will need to pay attention to internal factors such as body shape, muscle activation, joint position, and coordination of limbs. At the same time, you also need to pay attention to the external environment – gravity, ground reaction force (the force between the ground and your body), the type of surface you train on, other people, as well as features such as walls, railings, benches etc.

Keeping a check on these environmental factors shouldn't be too challenging. However, if you are new to bodyweight training, this level of concentration may result in greater mental fatigue following a training session. As your training experience increases, so too will your ability to maintain awareness of your environment.

EQUIPMENT

While the aim of this book is to present bodyweight training in as pure a form as possible, it's still important to have an appreciation of the scope that additional equipment can provide, as well as the potential for progression (and regression) it can offer to your training. Here are a few equipment options that can be added to any bodyweight training programme, some of which are used within this book.

- **Gymnastic rings** are growing in popularity as a mainstream fitness tool, thanks to the growing popularity of adult gymnastics in general, and to fitness training philosophies, such as CrossFit. The rings demand a high level of upper-body strength and stability, and advanced exercises, such as the muscle-up or iron cross, also require use of the false grip.

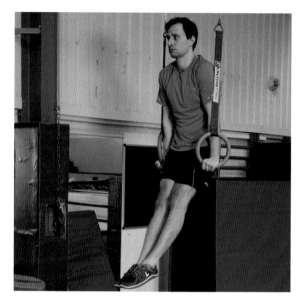

Figure 2.3a Gymnastic rings

- **Bars** including chin-up/pull-up bars as well as high bars, are used for a number of pulling movements. In contrast to the rings, the bars are fixed, and therefore demand less stabilisation. Entire bodyweight fitness routines can be performed on the bars, as popularised by the likes of the Bartendaz and Barstarzz fitness programmes.

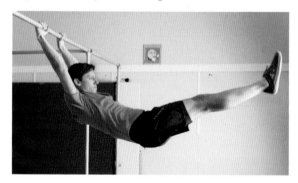

Figure 2.3b High bars/chin up bar/infinity rig

- **Parallel bars** are another staple piece of apparatus in men's artistic gymnastics. As a training tool, they offer many variations of pressing and pulling movements, as well as a number of abdominal/core exercises. Although P-bars are not common in modern fitness facilities, they are often found in many playgrounds and trim trails. When training indoors, parallettes can be used (or made), which offer a portable solution for training.

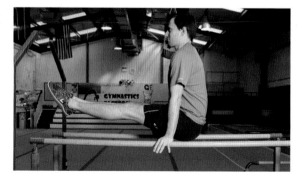

Figure 2.3c Parallel bars and parallettes

- **Suspension training systems** are a highly effective addition to any bodyweight training arsenal, and consist of two straps (with handles) attached to a high anchor point. In contrast to the rings, at least one leg is anchored to the floor, which provides added stability and reduces the amount of bodyweight pressed or pulled. In addition, exercises are quickly progressed/regressed by changing the position of the body, which affects the angle of pull.

- **Climbing ropes** are another example of a classic piece of equipment that has enjoyed a revival as a serious fitness tool. Much of their popularity has arisen from the boom in military fitness programmes, combined with the fact that fitness climbing ropes are highly portable – they can be carried in a rucksack and hooked around a tree or climbing frame – and are relatively cheap to buy.

- **Stability balls** have been in wide use in fitness training since the mid-1980s, having previously been used exclusively in physical therapy for many years. As well as providing a challenging unstable environment for training, they also allow the body to be used as an effective lever on the ball, e.g. during a push-up with the feet on the ball, the exercise is easier when the ball is closer to the hands, and become harder when the ball is closer to the feet.

- **Outdoor environments** contain an almost limitless array of equipment options that can be incorporated into an outdoor bodyweight training session – and are free to use. These include park benches, picnic tables, playgrounds, trim trails, walls, railings, and trees, to name a few.

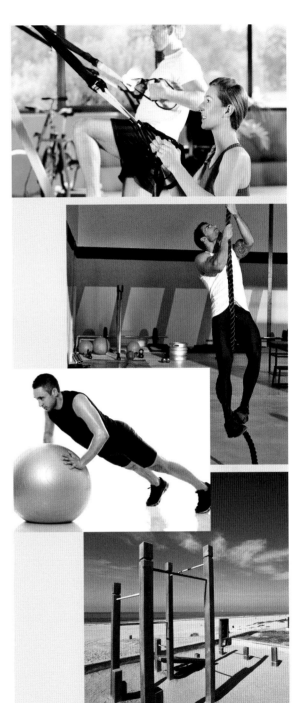

// TRAINING FORMATS

3

INTRODUCTION

For many bodyweight purists, the primary focus of training will be acquiring skills and transferring them to more complex activities. However, for those new to this type of training or those who are using bodyweight exercises alongside other forms of training, some more common objectives may apply. These may include increasing fitness, building muscle, core conditioning, improving strength, or weight loss.

As with any form of training, these objectives will depend on manipulation of acute exercise variables (as well as optimal recovery and sensible nutrition). To meet these objectives, several training formats are briefly discussed below which demonstrate the flexibility, diversity and scalability that bodyweight training has to offer. Please note that this is not an exhaustive list of training formats, however they have been designed to provide a starting point for those new to bodyweight training, as well as offer an avenue for further exploration by experienced individuals. Regardless of the training approach used, skilful movement should be prioritised to maximise training outcomes and minimise the risk of over-exertion and injury.

Each of the workouts falls into one of the following formats:

- General fitness and conditioning
- Metabolic conditioning
- Biomotor skill-based
- Movement skill-based
- Play/exploratory-based
- Task orientated.

Tip

Sample workout plans for each training format can be found in the appendix. The workouts cover a number of objectives, across various training methods and systems. The adoption of a particular training system or workout will depend on your bodyweight objectives (e.g. increasing fitness, skill acquisition, weight loss, etc.) as well as other factors, such as availability of time, space and equipment, and recovery from other training.

GENERAL FITNESS AND CONDITIONING WORKOUTS

These workouts are ideally suited to beginners, or those using bodyweight training secondary to another primary form of training. These sessions will often employ simple horizontal loading techniques (e.g. 3 sets of 10 reps) across a diverse range of exercises and biomotor skills. For specific outcomes, body regions can be targeted, e.g. whole body, lower body, upper body and core.

METABOLIC CONDITIONING WORKOUTS

Metabolic conditioning workouts aim to hit multiple energy systems within a single (shorter) session, resulting in high levels of energy expenditure and rapid fitness gains. As such, they are suitable for those who have a good level of fitness and/or training experience. These workouts commonly employ a circuit format that uses high-intensity interval training (HIIT) principles, e.g. timed or repetition circuits, Tabata cycles, etc.

High-intensity interval training (HIIT)

Many independent studies since the 1980s have confirmed that high-intensity interval training (HIIT) can have a much higher return on effort, compared to steady-state training methods. There is no specific recipe to HIIT, however a common approach involves a 2:1 ratio of work to recovery periods, e.g. 40 seconds of all-out exercise with 20 seconds recovery. Because of the higher intensities involved, HIIT sessions generally last no longer than 20–30 minutes.

Of particular interest in recent times has been the Tabata Protocol, created by Professor Izumi Tabata in Japan. It is a scientifically proven high-intensity interval training system that uses 20 seconds of ultra-intense exercise followed by 10 seconds of rest, repeated continuously for 4 minutes (8 cycles in total).

In the original study, athletes using this protocol trained four times per week, and obtained similar gains to a group of athletes who did steady state training (70% VO_2max) 5 times per week. The steady state group did have a higher VO_2max at the end of the study, but the Tabata group had started lower and gained more overall; they also showed improvements in anaerobic capacity (Tabata et al, 1996).

The original Tabata protocol is outlined below:
- 5 minutes of warm-up
- 8 intervals of 20 seconds all-out intensity exercise followed by 10 seconds of rest in between each interval (a timer is recommended)
- 2 minutes cool-down.

This protocol can be applied to any form of training, but is particularly suited to bodyweight training as it requires no equipment and can be performed almost anywhere.

BIOMOTOR SKILL-BASED WORKOUTS

These workouts are designed to improve a specific biomotor skill at any level of fitness. Biomotor skills (or abilities) can simply be thought of as the fundamental components of fitness, and include strength, power, endurance, speed, flexibility and agility. For example, a plyometric bodyweight workout may employ explosive movements, such as jumps, to build power; a higher repetition/timed circuit using whole body exercises, such as squats, push-ups or burpees, can be used to develop muscular endurance and cardiorespiratory fitness; and a programme that focuses on holding specific body shapes, such as supports, will help to develop correct body tension patterns and increase isometric strength.

MOVEMENT SKILL-BASED WORKOUTS

These programmes can be used to develop specific movement patterns either for general fitness or for athletic performance. The objective of movement skill training is the attainment of fluidity and control of movement with economy of effort. These workouts will often involve a progressive approach that involves breaking down a particular skill and drilling each component, before building them back into the skill, for example, drilling individual exercises towards the attainment of an unsupported handstand. Lower repetitions are used but often over multiple sets in order to minimise fatigue and groove optimal motor patterns. As confidence and technique improves, multiple skills can be trained within a single workout.

PLAY-/EXPLORATORY-BASED WORKOUTS

Play-based exercise represents an unstructured approach to training that is growing in popularity. This type of training has its roots in motor development, as well as the observations of distinct patterns of play in humans and other animals. This approach to developing fitness has undoubtedly been influenced by the philosophies and methods of dance, martial arts, and Parkour, as well as a number of somatic education formats.

What is somatic education?

Somatic education is an umbrella term for mind-body learning approaches that are kinaesthetic and somatosensory in nature, where movement and awareness are taught as a way to restore intuitive, natural movement. Such approaches are often very gentle and non-invasive, yet elicit change quickly. Common formats include the Feldenkrais Method, Hanna Somatics, Aston Patterning, and the Alexander Technique.

The fundamental aim of these sessions is exploratory, mindful movement, fuelled by a sense of wonder and curiosity. Each workout may explore just a few movements or may involve a continuous flow of movement using multiple exercises and sequences. This approach shifts the attention of training away from the attainment of sets and reps, allowing you instead to focus on body awareness and your immediate environment.

Play-based workouts can be very structured and goal oriented, or can be relaxed and spontaneous. The objective is to explore where to go from each start position, and how to fluidly link each successive movement using any other building block or locomotor movements. As you get a feel for this workout, use it to inspire other workouts of a similar nature. Note that the concept of sets and reps does not apply in these workouts.

TASK-ORIENTATED WORKOUTS

Task-orientated exercise is considered by many natural movement purists to be true functional training. The underlying premise for this approach is that in a natural or evolutionary context, sets and reps have no meaning – evolution only cares about your capacity to adapt and complete a given task.

In these types of workouts, a particular physical goal or task is set that requires the use of various bodyweight movements to complete. For example, in its simplest sense, this may involve the goal of getting from one side of a studio to the other; to add complexity, you could position obstacles in the way, only use crawling movement patterns, and set yourself a time limit. This type of training adds a higher level of psychological stress that will demand a continuum of physical skills – both orthodox and improvised – and the ability to quickly and efficiently strategise movement to complete the task in the most efficient way possible.

Task-orientated workouts can be fun, different, and experimental – and will often require a trial-and-error approach. With this in mind, their spontaneous nature makes them challenging to prepare and document, however, here are a few ideas that you can try, which may inspire further explorations.

- **Working out at home** – move between each room of your house using a different locomotor pattern (e.g. prone crawl, crab walk, hopping etc.). Set a physical task for each room, which must be completed before leaving the room (e.g. a 60-second isometric hold; 20 burpees; move from one end of your room to the other without putting your feet on the floor). If you have stairs, try crawling up (and down) them. For an additional challenge, include your garden.

- **Working out in an exercise studio** – set up various obstacles, e.g. steps of different heights, stability balls, cones, hurdles, exercise mats etc. Your objective is to navigate all obstacles without disrupting the flow of movement. If you pause at any point, you have to start from the beginning. For added motivation, use a timer.

- **Working out in the playground** – find a suitable playground (preferably when it's not busy!). Set yourself a goal of navigating the playground using as many appropriate movement patterns as possible. Your objective is to make contact with every piece of equipment. Once again, try not to pause as you move, and use a timer to motivate you.

- **Running through the woods/trails** – set yourself some objectives before you start your run. For example, every time you see a log either jump over it or dive forward roll, walk along it (balance), or even lift it several times, if possible; when you see a tree with a low hanging (strong) branch, hang from it or perform some pull-ups; if you see a suitable tree, climb it; vault over railings and walls, or walk along them; perform quadrupedal movements along the way (especially useful up steeper banks, or when the ground is softer/flatter). Integrating these bodyweight movements with your run will add plenty of unpredictability to your session, making it extremely challenging. And don't forget – you can add almost any bodyweight exercise or movement at any time during your run.

WARMING UP

4

The purpose of a warm-up is to prepare the body for the task(s) ahead. When starting exercise, the body will need to make a number of adjustments, including increases in heart and breathing rate, increases in metabolism, and increases in blood flow to working muscles (to supply oxygen and remove waste products). These adjustments do not occur straight away, and often take several minutes, and so the warm-up encourages these adjustments to occur gradually, by beginning exercise at a lower level of intensity and progressively increasing it.

The pre-exercise warm-up:

- increases blood flow to the muscles, which increases delivery of oxygen and nutrients
- warms the muscles, preparing them for increase in range of motion
- prepares the musculoskeletal and cardiorespiratory systems for an increase in activity
- primes neuromuscular pathways, ready for exercise
- provides mental preparation for the workout.

There are a number of options and techniques available for warming up before exercise, including body rolling, joint mobility, static and dynamic stretching, muscle-activation techniques, balance and stability exercises, and cardiorespiratory activities. While any of these warm-ups can be performed in isolation, in the interests of bodyweight training, an integrated warm-up that combines the above elements is strongly recommended. Not only will such an approach meet the multiple biomotor demands of bodyweight training, it will also effectively warm up the entire neuro-musculoskeletal system in a short space of time. With this in mind, the following sequence of activities is recommended as part of a structured warm-up:

1. Foot/ankle mobility
2. Neuromuscular activation
3. Dynamic mobilisation
4. Cardiorespiratory exercise.

It's also important to remember that any singular warm-up exercise or technique can be expanded if necessary. For example, when warming up for a workout that focuses on handstand progressions, more time should be spent on mobilising the shoulder joints and wrists as part of the overall warm-up. In addition, many of the bodyweight exercises in this book can be scaled down in volume and intensity, and subsequently be performed as part of a warm-up – this may be especially useful when training specific skills. For example, the front/side/back support exercises can be used in any warm-up to drill proper shape for more advanced exercises such as push-ups, handstands or cartwheels; deep squats and simple cadence jumps are also an excellent way to warm up for running.

FOOT/ANKLE MOBILITY

Almost every bodyweight exercise or skill will involve the foot making contact with the ground. To maximise the feedback from the ground to the foot, a strong yet mobile foot and ankle is required. If bodyweight training is to be performed in bare feet or wearing appropriate barefoot shoes, it's important to warm up the feet and ankles prior to exercise.

There are a number of simple, effective methods that can be performed as part of a warm-up including toe strengthening, ankle mobility techniques, and foot rolling – all of which will improve mobility, strength and proprioception (sensory feedback) in the feet and ankles. It's worth noting that long-term use of inappropriate footwear can predispose the toes, feet and ankles to immobility, soft tissue tightness/shortness and reduced strength – therefore restoration of these functions and improved proprioception through the use of these exercises may take some time.

The following exercises can be performed as part of a warm-up for any training session that is performed in bare feet. The exercises are designed to wake up the feet and allow them to become more responsive to some of the more challenging bodyweight skills that actively involve the feet. They may also be used as part of an ongoing corrective exercise programme to restore natural function in the feet and ankles following months and years of tension developed through the use of inappropriate footwear and poor exercise habits.

Perform the exercises in the order below, spending 30–60 seconds on each one.

Barefoot shoes and bodyweight training

The decision to go purely barefoot during bodyweight training will be a matter of preference, and one that is dependent on the training surface and terrain. However, sensory feedback is the foundation of skill, and to ensure maximum feedback, going barefoot is highly recommended.

When weather or terrain demands footwear, use of an appropriate barefoot shoe is advised. The perfect shoe will allow the foot to behave as if bare, while providing maximum protection from the environment.

With this in mind, the shoe should allow for sensory feedback from the ground via the sole; it should also protect your foot, which is especially relevant when performing exercise outdoors; and the shoe should follow the anatomy of the foot, providing enough room for the toes to spread forwards and outwards on impact. Meeting these requirements in shoe choice will allow for better performance and progression during bodyweight training, and will also strengthen your feet and ankles in the process.

STANDING

The simple act of standing is almost always taken for granted. For the most part, being well grounded in a standing position is a product of optimal proprioception between the plantar surface of the feet and the ground. Maximising this proprioception will not only improve reactivity to ground reaction forces during movement, but will subsequently optimise distribution of these forces through the lower extremity, thereby reducing the risk of injury. Standing with skill requires optimal strength, mobility and control of the big toe, which will then serve as a solid foundation for movement.

Stand with feet hip width apart, and toes pointing outwards approximately 10-15° – this should be a comfortable position, so feel free to adjust as necessary. Keep the shoulders relaxed and eyes facing forwards. As you stand, try to get a feel for where your weight is distributed – forward to back, and left to right. Visualise your heels and the balls of your feet, and aim to distribute your weight evenly between both; think about your weight from left to right foot and find a central point of balance.

Once you have a sense of balance, focus on the toes. The axis of balance in standing is between the second and third toes – visualise a straight line that passes through this point and the middle of your heel. At the same time, firmly (but not forcibly) push your big toe into the ground. The other toes should remain relaxed, in light contact with the ground.

Exercise 4.1 Big toe down

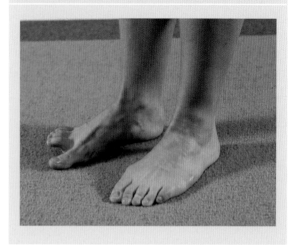

- In a standing position, push the big toe down into the floor and raise the other four toes off the floor
- As this can be extremely challenging at first, aim for small pulses of the movement
- Keep the ball of the foot in contact with the ground at all times, i.e. do not roll the foot inwards in order to lift the other four toes
- When your proprioception starts to improve, aim to hold the other four toes off the floor while pushing down the big toe for up to 30 seconds

Exercise 4.2 Big toe under

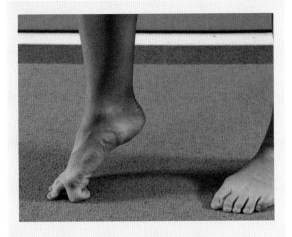

Exercise 4.3 Big toe forward

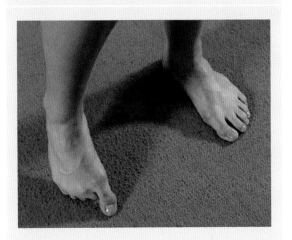

- With or without assistance, bend the big toe underneath the foot
- This can be an uncomfortable movement (often with restricted range of motion) so it's important to use a soft surface when doing this exercise
- It is important that the emphasis is on mobility at the first metatarsal joint. When viewed from above, it will appear as though the big toe has been chopped off at the metatarsal head

- With or without assistance, bend the four smaller toes underneath the foot, leaving the big toe pointing forwards
- In this position, push the big toe into the floor to improve strength in this position
- The bending of the toes can be uncomfortable (often with restricted range of motion) so it's important to use a soft surface when doing this exercise
- The emphasis should be on mobility at the metatarsal heads – when viewed from above, it will appear as though the smaller toes have been chopped off

Exercise 4.4 Toe stretch

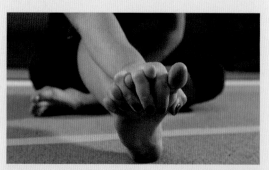

(a)

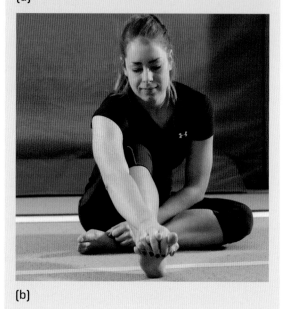

(b)

Exercise 4.5 Ankle mobility

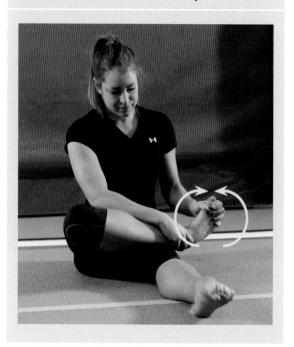

- In a seated or standing position, point the toes away from the body (plantar flexion), and then towards the body (dorsi flexion)
- Repeat several times slowly
- Take hold of the lower leg, and rotate the ankle in both directions several times

- In a seated position, interlace your fingers between your toes
- This stretches the muscles of the toes and allows them to spread
- Note that this action can be very challenging for some people due to wearing confining shoes

Exercise **4.6** Heel sit (dorsi flexion)

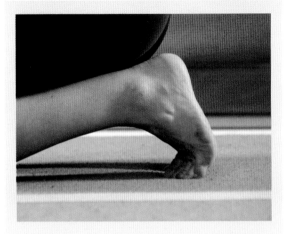

Exercise **4.7** Heel sit (plantar flexion)

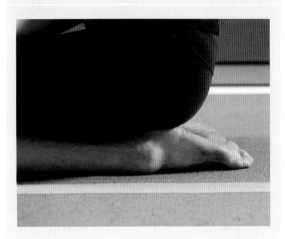

- In a kneeling position with the toes facing forwards, sit back on the heels, allowing the plantar surface of the feet to stretch
- Once in a relaxed position, push or pulse the big toes into the floor repeatedly allowing the body to gently rock back and forth
- In the same position, place your hands on your heels and slowly extend the hip and thoracic spine as you straighten your arms
- Once in this fully extended position, pulse the big toes as before, rocking the body back and forth

- Sit on the heels once more, except this time, plantar flex the ankle allowing the toes to face behind you – this time you will feel the stretch on the front of the ankle/foot
- As you settle into this position, gently lean back (supported by your hands) as far as is comfortable – feeling the stretch through the quads/hip flexors
- Take care not to overstretch in this position

Exercise 4.8 Foot rolling

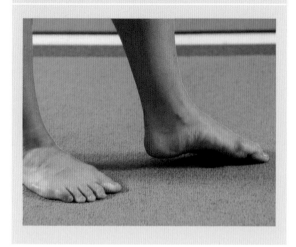

- Using a tennis ball or small rubber ball, roll along the entire sole of the foot
- Start from the base of the big toe and slowly roll along the inside of the foot towards the heel
- Do the same for the middle of the sole, and finally for the outside of the sole
- This helps to warm up the feet as well as relieving any tension in the intrinsic foot muscles

NEUROMUSCULAR ACTIVATION

Neuromuscular activation is an important stage of any warm-up, and consists of basic muscle-activation exercises that help to wake up the communication lines between the nervous system and the muscular system to prepare the body for activity.

Each muscle-activation exercise focuses on a low-level isometric contraction – no more than 25% of maximal voluntary effort for 6–10 seconds – which is just enough to facilitate activation of the muscle group. Each exercise is performed 2 to 3 times, with the entire sequence taking only 3 to 5 minutes.

The following muscle-activation sequence consists of 8 exercises, and should be performed at the start of a warm-up for bodyweight training. Please note that these are just a few examples of the many activation exercises available, and the reader is encouraged to explore these through further reading.

What is the right level of muscle activation?

In nature, creating the right level of muscle contraction for any given movement is not usually a conscious act, but one that is automatic and energy efficient. We learn the right levels during infancy and early childhood, but this knowledge is lost in adulthood if not maintained.

As we reconnect with bodyweight movements, it can be useful to set an initial reference level of intensity when it comes to muscle-activation exercises, often no more than about 25% maximum voluntary effort. The best way to do this in the first instance is to contract your muscles using maximum effort (i.e. 100%). Then do the same for half that (50%); finally do the same for half that (around 25%). Learn what this level of effort feels like, and practise this until you can do this consistently during the muscle-activation exercises. Remember that the objective is to activate or 'wake up' the muscles, not fatigue them.

As you practise bodyweight exercises, you'll begin to unconsciously activate muscles at the right level for any given movement, and usually this will decrease to a minimum as your skill increases.

Exercise 4.9 Standing hollow

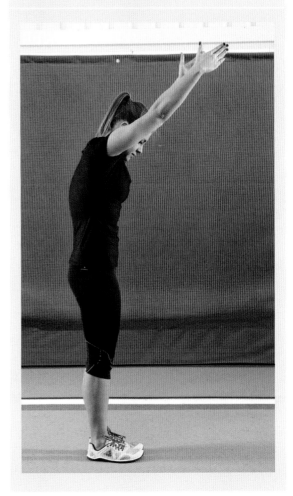

- Stand with feet together and arms straight overhead
- Engage the abdominals, glutes and quads
- This muscle effort will pull your body into a slight concave or hollow shape
- Hold for 6–10 secs, and repeat

Exercise **4.10** Front scale

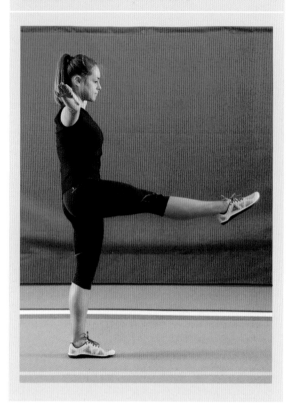

Exercise **4.11** Back scale

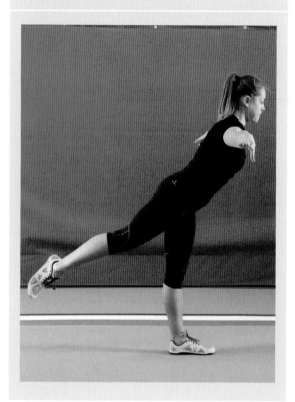

- Stand with feet together and arms straight out to the sides
- Engage the abdominals, glutes and quads, forming a hollow shape with the body
- Holding this shape, raise one leg up in front of you, keeping it straight
- Hold for 6–10 secs, and switch legs

- Start in the same position as the front scale
- Raise one leg straight behind you as you lean the torso forwards. There should be a straight line with the torso and back leg
- Hold for 6–10 secs, and switch legs

Exercise **4.12** Side scale

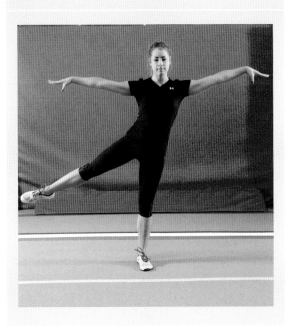

- Start in the same position as the front scale
- Raise one leg straight out to the side, keeping the glutes and quads engaged on both legs
- Hold for 6–10 secs, and switch legs

Exercise **4.13** Back support

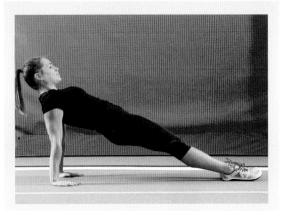

- In a seated position on the floor with legs straight out in front of you, place the hands just behind the hips, fingers pointing to the sides or backwards
- Push the arms straight into the floor as you drive the hips and chest upwards into a back support position
- Keep the glutes and quads engaged
- Hold for 6–10 secs

Exercise 4.14 Front support

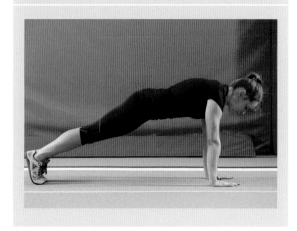

- Assume a push-up position with hands shoulder-width apart
- Engage the abdominals, glutes and quads, forming a hollow body shape
- Hold for 6–10 seconds

DYNAMIC MOBILISATION

Dynamic mobilisation exercises consist of slow controlled movements performed through a full range of motion. Following neuromuscular activation, these exercises will begin to warm soft tissue and increase extensibility, promote further muscle-activation patterns appropriate to training, and raise heart rate gradually.

Each exercise should be performed deliberately and rhythmically, with 4–6 repetitions per exercise. Aim to move smoothly from one exercise to the next without pausing. The following mobilisation sequence takes about 10 minutes to complete. If a shorter warm-up is required, simply select the relevant exercises. Dynamic mobilisation can also be structured into a standalone workout, which can be performed regularly alongside other bodyweight training. This can help to maintain or improve joint and soft tissue health, as well as support recovery from intensive training sessions.

Where muscles feel particularly stiff or exhibit limitations in range of motion, mobilisation exercises can be repeated several times; alternatively, body-rolling techniques are recommended to free up the soft tissues to enhance mobility. Several body-rolling exercises are explored as part of the cool down using a ball and foam roller – please refer to pages 55–59 for further details.

Exercise 4.15 Deep squat

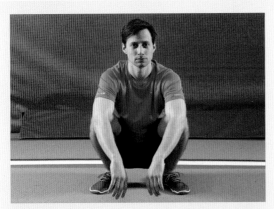

(a)

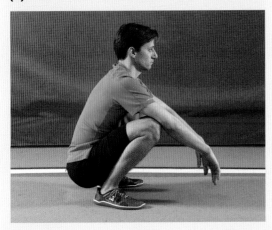

(b)

Improving range of motion in the deep squat

It's worth noting that the deep bodyweight squat is a natural human movement, first mastered in early childhood. Unfortunately, prolonged sitting, poor footwear and non-functional exercise prescription has made this simple, healthy exercise hugely challenging for the majority of adults, as they simply don't have the required range of motion. However, getting deep into the squat can be enhanced in several ways.

Raising the heels slightly by an inch can help to get deeper and allow your brain to learn what it feels like to squat deep; as your range improves, gradually reduce the heel lift. Alternatively, fear of falling backwards can also prevent people from performing the exercise properly. In this case, simply hold on to a bar or sturdy object in front of you as you squat. Keep the arms at full length as you do, and relax into the movement, bouncing lightly at the bottom to gently increase your range of motion. Using both of these simple techniques will allow your squat to deepen quickly and easily, opening up the potential for further movement skill.

- From a relaxed standing position, squat down as far as possible, reaching the hands towards the floor in front of you
- Aim to bring the hips as close to the floor as possible
- Return to standing and repeat

Exercise 4.16 Deep squat – hip in

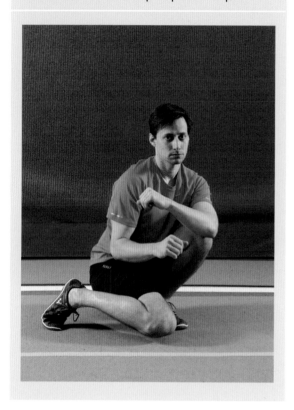

Exercise 4.17 Deep squat – hip out

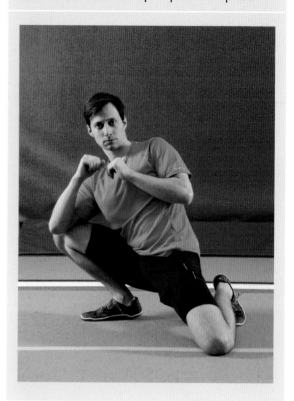

- Sit in a deep squat position
- Shift your weight across to one leg and rotate the opposite hip and knee in towards the floor
- Allow the torso to rotate as you do this
- Alternate from side to side

- Sit in a deep squat position
- Drive one hip forwards allowing the knee to touch the floor in front of the body. To help this motion, allow the opposite foot to slide outwards and the torso to rotate.
- Alternate from side to side

Exercise 4.18 Deep squat – short post and overhead reach

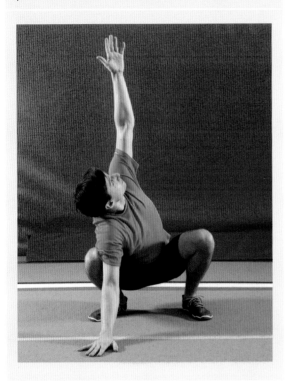

Exercise 4.19 Deep squat – long post and backwards reach

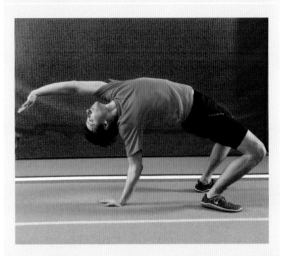

- Sit in a deep squat position
- Slide one hand on the floor and plant it approximately 12–15 inches behind the hip.
- Push this hand into the floor as you extend the hips upwards (table position) and reach the opposite hand over the body towards the floor
- Slowly return and repeat on the other side

- Sit in a deep squat position
- Place one arm inside the knee with the hand on the floor
- As you push the elbow into the knee, reach the opposite arm overhead, allowing the torso to rotate
- Pause in this position, before switching sides

Exercise 4.20 Lunge – forward reach

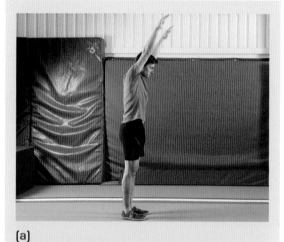

(a)

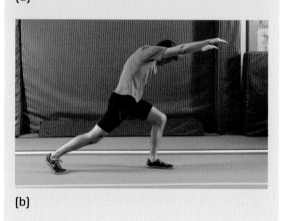

(b)

Exercise 4.21 Push-up plus

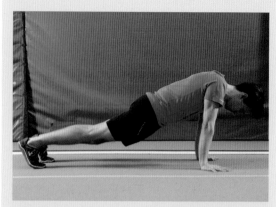

(a)

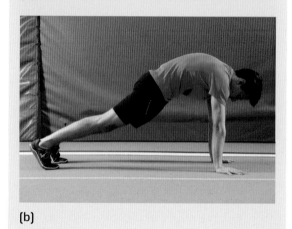

(b)

- In a standing position, straighten the arms overhead, engage the abdominals, and tuck in the chin
- Lunge forward on one leg, flexing the spine and reaching the arms forwards – as if casting a fishing rod
- Return and repeat on the other leg

- Assume a push-up/front support position, engaging the abdominals, glutes and quads
- Keeping the arms locked, push the hands into the floor and protract the shoulder blades – think about lifting the chest upwards. Feel the shoulder blades move apart
- Return to the start position, and allow your bodyweight to sink the chest further down to passively retract the shoulder blades
- Repeat several times

Exercise **4.22** Front support to downward-facing dog

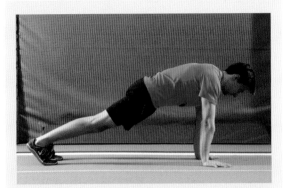

(a)

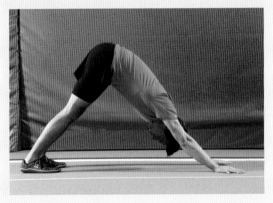

(b)

Exercise **4.23** Spinal rock

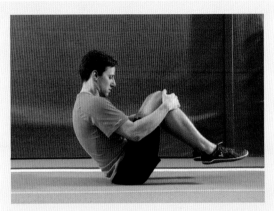

(a) Shoulder position

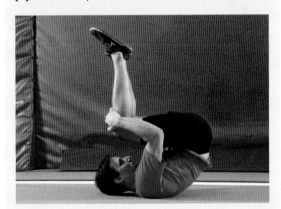

(b) Low back position

- From the front support position, keep the arms and legs straight as you push the hips up and back into an inverted-V position (in yoga known as a downward-facing dog)
- Pause momentarily before returning to front support

- Lying on your back on an exercise mat or soft surface, hold your knees into your chest, and tuck in the chin
- Roll backwards and forwards gently across your spine while holding this tucked position

CARDIORESPIRATORY EXERCISE

The final phase of the warm-up is cardiorespiratory exercise, the aim of which is to increase heart rate and blood flow to meet the demands of the exercise session. Almost any aerobic exercise will be suitable, however, in the spirit of true bodyweight training, the following 6 exercises have been chosen.

Each exercise should be performed for 30–60 secs, with minimal rest between exercises. This part of the warm-up should take 3–5 minutes to complete.

Exercise 4.24 Plyometric bounces

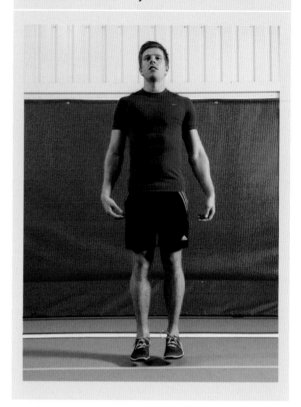

- Bounce on the balls of your feet at a fast pace – if a metronome is available, set it to 180 bpm and bounce in time to this tempo
- Allow the shoulders, arms and wrists to relax as you bounce
- As a variation, perform opposite hip and torso rotations at the same pace

Exercise 4.25 Running heel pulls

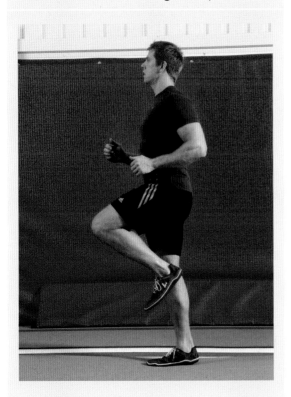

Exercise 4.26 Jumping jacks

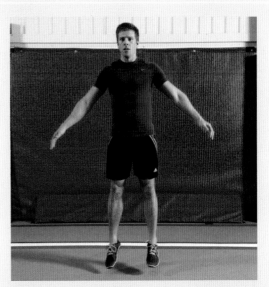

(a)

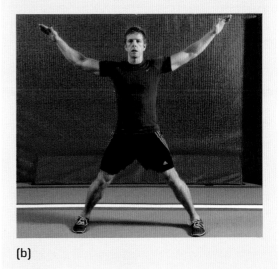

(b)

- Run on the spot and pull your heels up behind you as fast as possible
- If a metronome is available, set it to 180 bpm and pull the heels in time to this tempo

- From standing, jump the legs out to the side, while simultaneously swinging the arms out and overhead
- Jump back in and repeat continuously

Exercise 4.27 Deep squat bounces

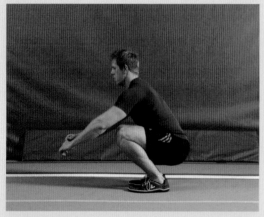

(a)

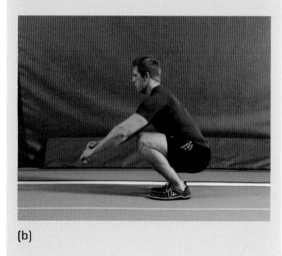

(b)

Exercise 4.28 Boxing combo

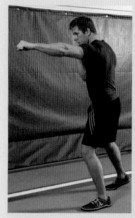

(a) Jab

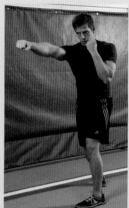

(b) Cross

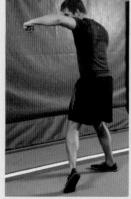

(c) Hook

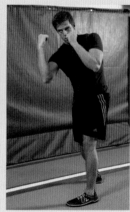

(d) Upper cut

- From standing, rapidly drop into a deep squat and bounce back up only part of the way
- Immediately drop down again and repeat continuously

- Assume a fighting stance, and perform the jab/cross/hook/upper cut combination several times
- Repeat on the other side

Sample warm-up sequence

The following table highlights a sample warm-up sequence for a bodyweight training session.

Exercise	Repetitions	Duration
Foot/ankle mobility		
Big toe down/under/ forward; toe stretch; ankle rotations	1 of each exercise	30 s each
Neuromuscular activation		
Standing hollow	3	6-10 s hold
Front scale	2 each leg	6-10 s hold
Back scale	2 each leg	6-10 s hold
Front support	3	6-10 s hold
Back support	3	6-10 s hold
Dynamic mobilisation		
Deep squat	4	
Deep squat – hip in	4 each side	
Deep squat – hip out	4 each side	
Deep squat – long post and backward reach	3 each side	
Lunge – forward reach	4 each side	
Front support to downward-facing dog	4	
Cardiorespiratory exercise		
Plyometric bounces		30-60 s
Running heel pulls		30-60 s
Jumping jacks		30-60 s
Boxing combo		30-60 s

// COOLING DOWN

5

The process of cooling down after exercise involves progressively slowing down your level of activity which:

- helps to restore heart rate and breathing to near resting levels
- helps avoid feelings of dizziness, which can result from blood pooling in the large muscles of the legs when intensive exercise is stopped suddenly
- helps to remove waste products (such as lactic acid) from muscles, which can build up during exercise
- helps to relax muscles, and prepare the body for the next exercise session.

An effective cooling down routine should last a minimum of 5–10 minutes, and should begin with a continuation of exercise while gradually lowering the intensity. This should then be followed by suitable soft tissue techniques that help to relax muscles, reduce stiffness, and restore/improve flexibility. Finally, flexibility techniques will help to restore and improve

muscle length. To meet these objectives, the following sequence of activities is recommended as part of a structured cool down. However, any of the previously described warm-up activities can also be performed, as long as the intensity is progressively scaled down in an appropriate manner.

1. Dynamic movement
2. Body-rolling techniques
3. Functional flexibility.

DYNAMIC MOVEMENT

The first part of the cool down is a continuation of exercise using simple whole body activities that promote movement of the arms and legs at progressively lower intensities. The aim is to bring the heart rate down and prevent blood pooling in the extremities. This process will also help to dissipate excess lactic acid build up in the muscles, and lower the rate of ventilation so that breathing returns to near normal. This part of the cool down should last for at least 3–5 minutes, and may include the following activities:

Exercise 5.1 Jumping jacks

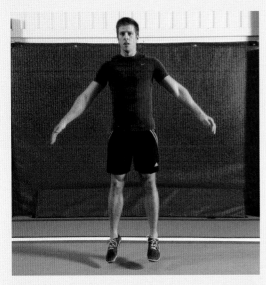

(a)

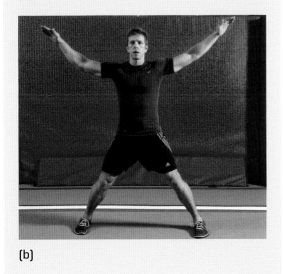

(b)

Exercise 5.2 Bouncing and shaking

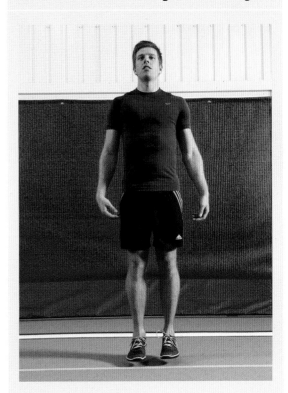

- Perform fast bouncing on the spot while shaking out the shoulders, arms and wrists
- For variety, add some alternate hip/torso twists

- Start at a faster pace, reducing this as you cool down

Exercise 5.3 Squat and lunge variations

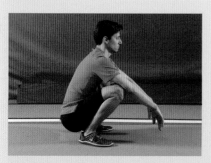

(a) Deep squat

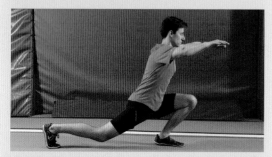

(b) Deep forward lunge

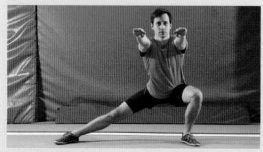

(c) Deep side lunge

- Perform several deep squats and deep lunges
- Add arm reaches and torso rotation to encourage range of motion in the shoulders and spine

BODY-ROLLING TECHNIQUES

Body-rolling techniques help to maintain the health of the neuromuscular system through self-massage. The technique commonly uses a ball or a foam roller. Whichever tool is chosen, rolling focuses on the neural (nerves) and fascial (connective tissue) systems that can be negatively influenced by poor posture, repetitive motions, or unskilful movements. These actions are recognised as an injury by the body, and can lead to inflammation, muscle spasm, and the development of soft-tissue adhesions. These adhesions can reduce elasticity of the soft tissues, eventually causing changes in the soft tissue structure that can affect movement. Rolling focuses on alleviating these adhesions to restore optimal joint motion and movement.

The technique involves a process of placing a ball or foam roller at the point where a muscle attaches to the bone. Your bodyweight is then allowed to sink into the ball/roller. The muscle is then rolled further by moving the body slowly along the ball/roller for 30–60 seconds to initiate further muscle release and fascial realignment.

Using a foam roller

The foam roller is by far the most common rolling tool, and is widely accessible in many forms. For most people a 12–15-inch-high density foam roller is recommended, such as the Grid™. The cylindrical shape of the roller makes it suitable for rolling the longer muscles such as the calves, hamstrings and spinal muscles.

Using a ball

Rolling with a ball is a less common, but highly effective technique. A 6–8-inch ball – such as a gymnastics ball – is an excellent choice in terms of size, and these balls can also be inflated or deflated to adjust the level of pressure required. The spherical shape is more suited to smaller muscles, as well as areas where multiple muscles converge, such as the glutes and back of the shoulder.

Several body-rolling techniques are detailed below, that may be useful during the cool-down phase of a bodyweight training session. For those wishing to explore this technique further, please refer to the recommended reading list at the back of this book.

Exercise 5.4 Calf foam ball

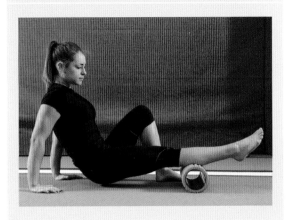

- In a seated position with legs straight and arms by your side, position a foam roller at the lower end of the calf on one leg
- Keep the other leg to the side
- Push the hands into the floor and lift the buttocks. Pause here for a few seconds, allowing your bodyweight to sink into the roller
- As you begin to relax, slowly roll up the calf towards the back of the knee. Move slowly over 30 secs. If necessary, add more pressure by placing the free leg on top of the rolling leg. For more coverage, roll up the inside and outside of the calf by slightly rotating the leg inwards or outwards, respectively

Exercise 5.5 Hamstrings

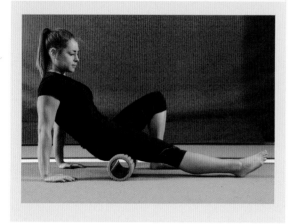

- In a seated position, with one leg straight and one bent, position a foam roller at the top of one hamstring, in the buttock crease
- Pause here for a few seconds as you allow your bodyweight to sink into the roller – use your hands and free leg for support
- Note that it may take a little longer for the tissues to begin to relax due to the mass of tendons at the top of the hamstrings
- As you begin to relax, slowly roll down the hamstrings towards the back of the knee. Move slowly over 30 seconds
- If necessary, add more pressure by placing the free leg on top of the rolling leg
- For more coverage, roll up the inside and outside of the hamstrings by slightly rotating the leg inwards or outwards, respectively

Exercise 5.6 Quadriceps

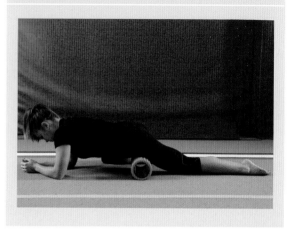

- Lie on your front, resting your weight on your forearms
- Place a foam roller at the top of one thigh in the hip crease – bend the free leg into a frog position
- As you begin to relax, slowly roll down the quads towards the knee. Move slowly over 30 seconds
- For more coverage, roll down the inside and outside of the quads by slightly rotating the leg outwards or inwards, respectively

Glute sequence

Exercise 5.7 Glute ball roll (sacrum)

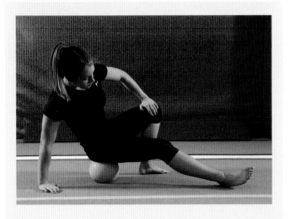

Exercise 5.8 Glute ball roll (pelvis)

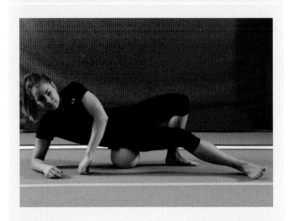

- This 3-minute sequence targets all areas of the glutes
- In a seated position with hands by your hips, place the ball at the base of the spine, just above the tail bone
- Bend one leg, placing the foot flat on the floor for support – this will be the non-rolling side
- Keep the other leg extended but slightly bent, resting on the heel
- Lean back on to the hands and rotate the torso/pelvis to the rolling side – you will feel the ball drop off the bony part of the spine and begin to press into the soft tissue of the gluteus maximus
- As you begin to relax, slowly roll across the glutes towards the hip bone, taking about 15–20 seconds to do so
- Lift off the ball and reposition higher up the sacrum, and repeat the roll along this new line
- Repeat a final time from the top of the sacrum

- Position the ball at the top of the pelvis on one side, and rotate the body towards the ball so that you are halfway towards being on your side
- You should feel the ball pressing into the fleshy part of the glutes – for comfort, you may wish to rest your bodyweight on the forearm of the same side. Allow your bodyweight to sink into the ball, then slowly begin to roll down the side of the glutes towards the greater trochanter. Once again, take 15–20 seconds, and repeat if necessary. Repeat this entire sequence on the other side of the body

Exercise 5.9 Thoracic spine foam roll

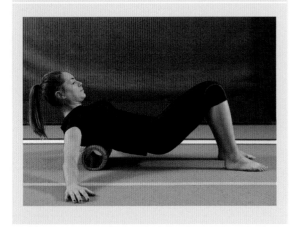

Exercise 5.10 Back of shoulders ball roll

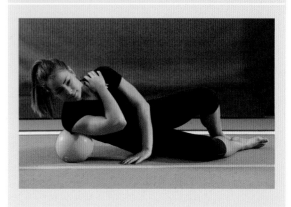

- A foam roller or ball can also be used on the thoracic spine
- Lie on your back with knees bent, and position the ball/roller at the base of the thoracic spine (just above the last ribs)
- Keep the head and hips raised off the ground and maintain a hollow body shape. The arms can remain on the floor by your sides, or support the head
- As the tissues begin to relax, slowly roll up the spine, taking 30-60 seconds – stop when you reach the top of the thoracic spine (base of neck)
- For more coverage, you can also roll up each side of the spine, by rotating the torso slightly

The area behind and underneath the shoulders is where a number of muscles converge that often exhibit stiffness and tightness following bodyweight training. Rolling out these areas with a ball will help to release tension.

- Begin by lying on your side, and place the ball underneath the shoulder and as far back as possible (without rolling off the ball)
- Use the hand of the rolling arm to grab the opposite shoulder – this will put a slight stretch on the shoulder as you roll
- Allow the ball to sink into the back of the shoulder for a few seconds, then slowly roll across the shoulder towards the elbow, taking about 15-20 seconds
- Aim to roll along the deltoid muscle, and also within the space between the rear deltoid and long head of the triceps

Exercise 5.11 Side of torso ball roll

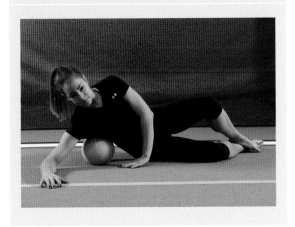

Another area that often requires releasing is the side of the upper torso, just below the armpit (serratus anterior and latissimus dorsi muscles).

- Lie on your side and position the ball just below the armpit. Because this region can be quite bony, you may wish to use a slightly deflated or softer ball
- Slowly and gently roll the ball backwards towards your shoulder blade for about 10 seconds – if you remain relaxed, you will feel the shoulder blade being pushed back towards the spine
- Repeat several times if necessary
- To release the latissimus dorsi muscle specifically, position the ball high in the armpit and slowly roll down the side of the torso, taking care to stay on the latissimus muscle and not to roll too far down on to the ribcage

FUNCTIONAL FLEXIBILITY

The traditional use of static stretching techniques in fitness programmes is controversial. While there is moderate evidence to indicate that regular stretching improves range of motion, strength and reduces injury risk, there is also evidence to suggest that acute pre-exercise (warm-up) stretching in isolation decreases strength and performance (Clark and Lucett, 2011).

However, the use of functional flexibility as part of a structured cool down can significantly restore tissue extensibility and reduce muscle tension, especially when performed immediately after body-rolling techniques.

The following flexibility techniques will help restore and improve flexibility in the major muscle groups, and build on the areas that were previously rolled. Each position should be held for 20–30 seconds and repeated as necessary. Please note that the technique of loading the body appropriately in each position is the key to success, and helps to differentiate between functional flexibility and traditional static stretching. To add an element of focus and flow to the routine, move from one position to the next in a fluid manner.

Exercise 5.12 Deep squat

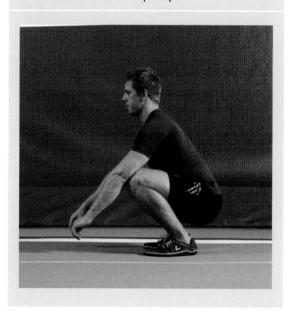

- From standing, slowly drop into a deep squat position and relax
- If you find it challenging to get deep enough, try holding onto a fixed object, such as a bar, and gently bouncing further into the deep squat position
- Alternatively, raise the heels by about an inch, which will allow you to drop deep into the squat

Exercise 5.13 Modified Chaturanga

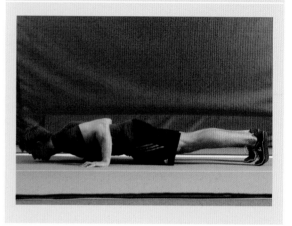

- From a deep squat position, reach the arms forward and assume a push-up position with fingers pointing out slightly
- Bend the elbows and keep them close to your sides, as you drop down as low as possible without the chest touching the floor
- Lean your bodyweight forwards over your hands and hold
- If this is too challenging, allow the knees and pelvis to rest on the floor as you continue to hold this position

Exercise 5.14 Modified upward-facing dog

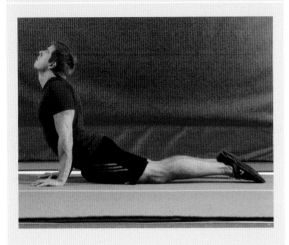

Exercise 5.15 Downward-facing dog

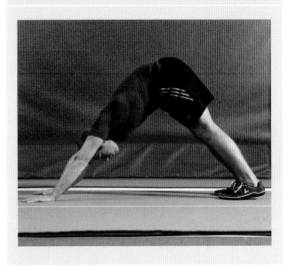

- From the modified Chaturanga position, push the hands into the floor and straighten the arms
- As you do this the chest will rise and the back will arch
- Lean your bodyweight forwards over your hands, and hold

- From the modified upward-facing dog position, keep your arms and legs straight as you drive the hips upwards and backwards into an inverted position
- Open up the shoulders, push the chest towards your feet, and hold

Exercise 5.16 Deep lunge

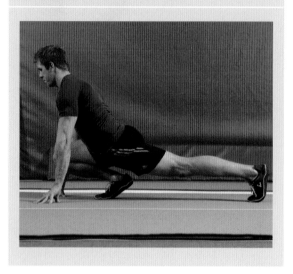

Exercise 5.17 Deep side lunge

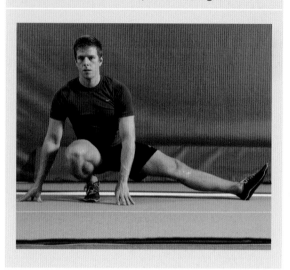

- From the downward-facing dog position, swing one leg through into a deep lunge position
- Place the hands on the floor as you lean your bodyweight as far forwards as possible over the front leg, keeping the back leg straight
- To allow you to put all your weight into the front leg, raise the heel so you are resting on the ball of the foot.
- Hold, and repeat on the other leg

- From the deep lunge position, pivot on the ball of the front foot into a side lunge position
- Keep your bodyweight as far over the bent leg as possible, and straighten the other leg out to the side with the toes pointing up
- Hold, before shifting your weight over and repeating on the other leg

Exercise 5.18 Deep glutes

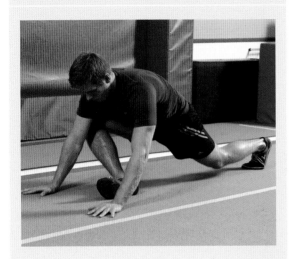

- From the side lunge, pivot back round to the forward lunge position and allow the front knee to drop out to the side
- Keep the back leg as straight as possible as you lean your weight as far forward as possible over the front foot (which will be turned out)
- Use your hands to support you as you drop the chest towards the foot
- Hold, before shifting your weight over and repeating on the other leg

Example cool-down session

The following table highlights a sample cool down sequence for a bodyweight training session.

Exercise	Repetitions	Duration
Dynamic movement		
Jumping jacks		I min
Bouncing and shaking		I min
Body rolling		
Calves (foam roller)		30 s each leg
Hamstrings (foam roller)		30 s each leg
Glutes (ball)		I min each side
Thoracic spine		I min
Functional flexibility		
Deep squat		20 s
Modified Chaturanga		20 s each leg
Modified upward-facing dog		20 s each leg
Downward-facing dog		30 s each side
Deep lunge		30 s each side
Deep side lunge		30 s each side
Deep glutes		30 s each side

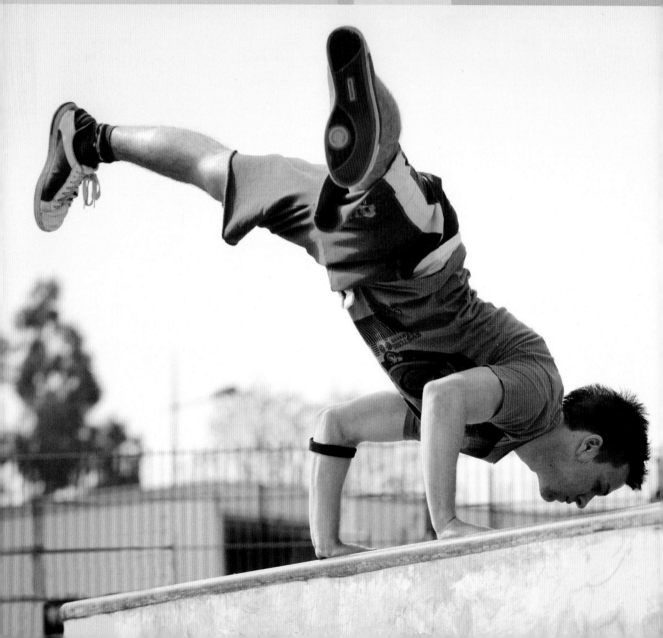

3

PART **THREE**

BODYWEIGHT SKILLS

This section focuses on fundamental bodyweight exercises and movements. These should be considered as the essential building blocks that make up higher skill movements and sequences. Many bodyweight enthusiasts are often motivated towards the higher skill exercises, but don't make that mistake – the importance of mastering these simple (yet challenging) building blocks cannot be overstated. Some of the highly skilful movement disciplines such as gymnastics, dance and martial arts are built on what is often a series of simple exercises and movements that are practised and drilled over months and years.

The exercises that follow are based on a motor developmental model of physical education, combined with basic principles of biomechanics that will allow for a systematic progression towards acquiring bodyweight skills. It's worth reminding ourselves that motor development has three important objectives:

1. To build sufficient **strength** to overcome gravity
2. To enable the body to **balance** under its base of support
3. To improve limb **coordination** for efficient movement.

In healthy humans, these objectives are achieved through the progressive development of three types of gross motor skills: stability skills, manipulative skills and locomotor skills. Within the context of bodyweight training, these gross motor skills provide a useful framework for physical development, which begins with simple static exercises before progressing towards more complex movement sequences.

Chapter 6, **Stability skills**, contains exercises that begin the development of strength and balance via simple isometric exercises that develop correct body shapes. A number of important static shapes are explored, as well as coordinated movement within these shapes. It's important to understand that the creation and maintenance of correct body shapes not only teaches proper muscle-activation patterns that can protect joints and preserve economy of effort, but can also provide a stable base during transition from one movement to another. Once a strong foundation of stability and balance has been built, chapter 7 on **Manipulative skills** explores ways to incorporate these skills into the two familiar patterns of pushing and pulling. Variations and progressions of these patterns are discussed to stimulate further adaptations in strength, balance and coordination, not only to promote skill development, but also to enhance the training effect. Chapter 8 on **Locomotor skills** provides progressions and imaginative variations on a number of locomotor patterns. While these patterns can be explored in parallel with stability and manipulative skills, many of the advanced locomotor skills (such as vaulting and rolling) require a strong foundation in stability; you may find that a regular revisit of the chapters on stability skills and manipulative skills will help you to master these skills.

The order of these exercise progressions is also important. Early motor learning is concerned with developing stability (and some manipulative skills) before more complex upright locomotor patterns develop. As adults, it makes sense to adopt a similar approach – bodyweight-based stability and manipulative skills will build a strong foundation for enhancing locomotor skills and more complex movement sequences. In practice, it's not necessary to master every movement before moving on to the next skill category; however, it's suggested that you master some of the basic shapes and positions before trying out some of the complex locomotor and movement sequences.

As your competency and confidence in these skills improves, there will be plenty of opportunity for further physical development. This can occur by playing around with the many variations and progressions of individual skills or through movement sequences, which involve combinations of the above skills. These movement sequences, or flows, are explored in the final section of the book and are hoped to encourage an experimental approach to bodyweight training.

STABILITY SKILLS 6

INTRODUCTION

Stability skills are motor skills involving balance or postural control, such as a single leg balance, or squat. They require maintaining one's centre of gravity over a base of support with minimal movement (static stability/balance), as well as the ability to perform a task while maintaining a stable position (dynamic stability/balance). These skills are among the first to develop in babies, and continue to serve as an important foundation for the correct execution of complex locomotor and manipulative movements during our physical development.

Natural human movement will often blur the boundaries of these definitions, resulting in combinations and sequences of static and dynamic stability that are unique to the task at hand. Unfortunately, technology and the demands of modern lifestyles can also detrain our ability to statically and dynamically stabilise our bodies, resulting in movement impairment, increased risk of injury, and pain. Therefore, there is a strong rationale to make stability skills an important part of our ongoing physical education.

In early childhood, stability is first developed as the body responds to gravity, allowing the head to be lifted and held in position. This is quickly followed by increased stability through the shoulder and pelvic girdle, arms and legs via pushing, pulling and crawling. As a child begins to experience upright posture through sitting and standing, gravity starts to shape stability in these positions. Eventually the child begins to integrate these stability patterns into important manipulative and locomotor skills.

Using this as a framework, stability can be improved in adults using similar exercise progressions that will effectively reboot these fundamental stability movements and enhance function in daily activities.

The following types of stability exercises will be explored in this section. Each group of exercises will begin with appropriate static stability drills, followed by suitable progressions and variations to dynamic movements, where applicable:

1. Floor-based supports
2. Double and single leg stability
3. Suspended supports
4. Hand balancing (advanced).

It's important to note that these stability exercises can form part of a general bodyweight fitness programme, as well as a specific conditioning programme for learning advanced bodyweight skills, such as handstands and muscle-ups. Throughout all the progressions, there is a common focus on developing good static control of body shape, as this allows for efficient transfer and distribution of force during complex movement skills and sequences.

Static exercises are usually held in a specific position for timed sets. With this in mind, planned progression should start in a manageable position before moving on to progressively harder positions as endurance improves. Bodyweight training should take full advantage of manipulating limb and body length to create not only a desirable position (and attain economy of effort) but also to challenge fitness. The more stable a joint is, the more force the neuromuscular system will allow to pass through that joint. If joint stability is less than optimal, the nervous system will lessen available power in an effort to protect the body.

FLOOR-BASED SUPPORTS

These exercises begin with simple flexion and extension body shapes, which are then progressed to a number of body-supported positions that are designed to build a foundation of static stability for advanced bodyweight skills. When practising these supports, there should be a strong focus on making the *correct* body shape, even if only for a few seconds. As strength and control improves, hold times should be increased up to 30–60 seconds.

The main outcome of drilling these positions is to improve the ability to hold a tight body position (also known as midline stability) during dynamic bodyweight movements, which in turn will significantly increase the transfer of force through from lower to upper body and vice versa. It's important to note that many of these positions involve supporting the upper body through the shoulders, arms and hands, consequently building high levels of stability in these positions; where applicable there will be an equal activation of the glutes, quads and calves to maintain and improve stability through the hips, knees and ankles.

Exercise 6.1 Hollow body hold

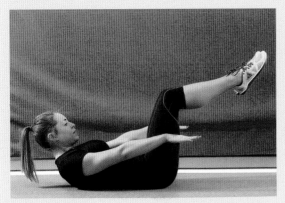
(a) Knees bent

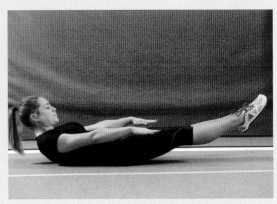
(b) Legs straight

Central to efficient transfer of force through the body is the maintenance and control of a hollow body – a shape that has significant crossover to other bodyweight movements. The ability to quickly and efficiently flex the body has safety implications, such as self-protection when falling, however, sustained control of extension is also important during longer duration activities, such as running. Having said that, while most individuals will be able to perform this simple movement over a short time, many will lack sustained control.

Basic movement

- In a lying supine position, bend the knees, flatten the back, and then raise the knees off the floor
- From here, tuck the chin in and hold this position while raising the head and shoulders off the floor
- When performed correctly, the eyes should be looking towards the pelvis
- As you become stronger, you can begin to raise the arms off the floor, reaching your fingertips past the feet, before progressing to arms reaching overhead
- As your ability to maintain this position improves, progressively straighten the legs. Note that the weight of the arms and legs will pose a significant flexion challenge for the trunk – your aim is to maintain a flat low back throughout
- Explore taking the arms overhead first before extending the legs. The arms should be straight (next to your ears) and the legs straight out between 6–12 inches off the ground
- Aim to reach with the arms and legs, rather than just lift them, maintaining the hollow shape throughout
- When you can perform the hollow with straight legs, begin grooving the correct muscle-activation patterns for retaining this shape by engaging the glutes and quadriceps

Progression: see exercise 6.2, hollow body rock

Exercise 6.2 Hollow body rock

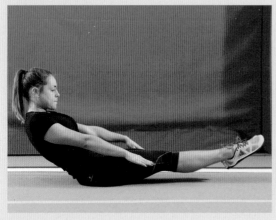

(a) Arms up

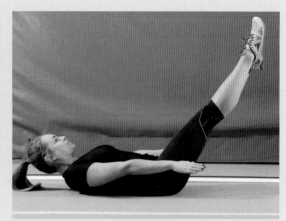

(b) Legs up

Although the attainment of a proper hollow hold is a transferable skill for other bodyweight movements, dynamic progressions such as this one will support skill development of a number of advanced bodyweight movements through further improvements in muscular endurance and control.

- Assume a fully extended hollow shape as before – maintain this position as you rock the entire body back and forth along your back

- This is an extremely challenging exercise, and the tendency to arch the back and lose the rocking motion will slow down progress initially. If this happens, rest a while, and then regress the exercise by tucking the legs in more, or reducing the range of rocking motion. The motion will eventually become smooth and uninterrupted, and can be progressed further by rocking faster.

Exercise **6.3** Seated balance

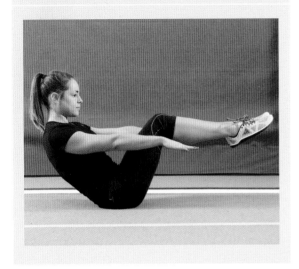

Exercise **6.4** Seated balance to roll

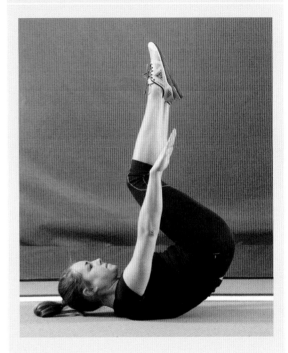

The seated balance is an excellent core exercise that involves both the trunk and hip flexors. Learning how to balance bodyweight over the hips in the seated position is also useful when transitioning into and out of rolling movements.

Basic movement

- In a seated position with hands by your side, bend the knees so that the feet are flat on the floor in front of you
- Engage the core, and lift the feet off the ground, tucking the knees into the chest
- Slowly raise the arms to horizontal and hold for 10–30 seconds

Progression: see exercise 6.4, seated balance to roll

The maintenance of a tight body shape (tuck) will allow you to execute the roll smoothly.

- From the seated balance position, maintain a tight hollow shape and roll backwards keeping the knees tucked and allowing the arms to reach overhead
- Keep the chin tucked so the head doesn't touch the floor
- Use the momentum to drive you back to the starting balance position
- Repeat as necessary

Exercise 6.5 Seated leg lift

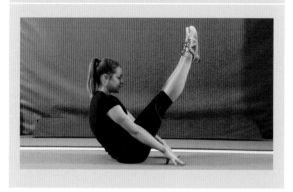

The seated leg lift is another highly effective core exercise. As a fundamental gymnastics drill, it will help to strengthen the abdominals as part of the L-sit progression.

Basic movement

This exercise places a high demand on trunk and hip flexor strength, as well as flexibility of the hamstrings. If these areas are limited, try leaning back slightly as you lift the legs – once the legs are up (even a couple of inches will do) flex the trunk hard and keep reaching the hands forwards.

- Sit on the floor with legs out straight and slide the arms forwards on the floor just above the knees
- Engage the core and quads, and raise the legs as far off the floor as you can, keeping them straight and together
- Push the hands into the floor to assist the leg lift, and use this pressing action to engage the scapular stabilisers – this is an important action to master for progressing on to the seat lift and L-sit
- Hold for several seconds, and slowly return to the start position

Exercise 6.6 Seat lift

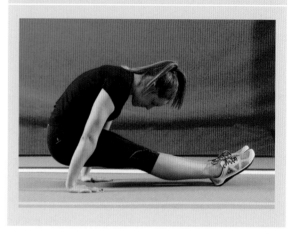

The seat lift is the opposing movement to the seated leg lift, and the other half of the progression towards the L-sit exercise.

Basic movement

- Sit on the floor with legs out straight and hands by your hips
- Engage the core and quads, and push the hands into the floor as you raise the hips
- Keep the trunk flexed over the hips and hold for several seconds, before returning to the start position

Maintaining a forward flexed trunk is key to balance and progression. As your abdominals become stronger, position your hands closer towards your knees – this will require you to flex the trunk hard and lean forwards into the hold to stay balanced. Gradually build up your hold times.

Exercise 6.7 Shoulder stand

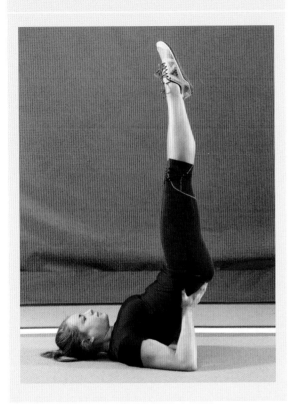

Basic movement

- Lie on your back with legs straight, toes pointed
- Bend the knees and bring them to your chest, keeping the arms on the floor by your sides for balance
- Rock back and forth a few times (hollow body roll) until you build enough momentum to roll back on to your shoulders
- As you do so, quickly push your hips up and straighten the legs towards the ceiling, creating a long, straight line from your hips to your toes
- Engage the glutes and quads, and hold momentarily
- Use your hands to support your mid-back region until you build sufficient strength in the abdominals to support your weight without them
- Release the hands, allow the hips to drop, bend the knees, and roll back down to the start position under control

The shoulder stand is an excellent conditioning exercise for developing strength and control in the trunk. It's also a useful prerequisite for the candlestick roll (pages 158–159) – a combination of the backward roll and shoulder stand.

Exercise 6.8 Front support (floor)

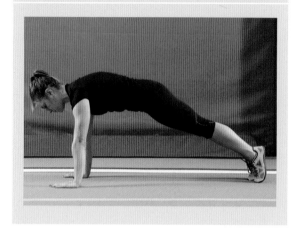

Exercise 6.9 Front support (lean)

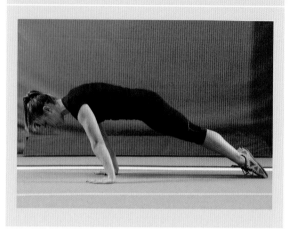

The prone front support is one of the most important bodyweight stability exercises to master and is hugely transferable to a number of other skills. In its purest form, it's simply a prone progression of the hollow body hold.

Basic movement
- Begin in a push-up position with hands underneath the shoulders
- Assume a hollow shape and maintain this by activating the glutes and quads
- The aim is to achieve the same degree of hollowing as with the hollow body hold
- Hold this position for 10–60 secs

Progression: see exercise 6.9, front support (lean)

Also known as the planche lean, this is a great drill for planche development. Please note that this is an extremely challenging exercise for the entire body.
- From the front support position, lean the body forwards taking the shoulders in front of the wrists
- To maintain balance and minimise stress on the wrists, you will need to increase tension in the hollow shape
- Advanced progressions involve elevating the legs, either on a step or in suspension

Exercise **6.10** Side support

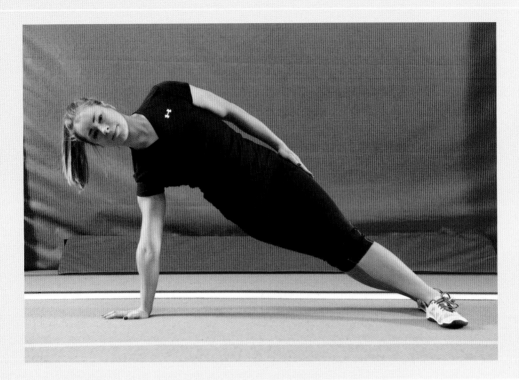

The side support offers a useful variation that should be included as part of a well-balanced conditioning programme. It's also an important body position in dynamic skills such as vaulting.

Basic movement
Due to the reduced base of support, this exercise will require higher levels of stability through the shoulder, trunk and hip.

- From the front support position, maintain the hollow shape as you rotate the entire body to the side support position; the top leg can rest on, or just in front of, the lower leg, and uppermost arm should be kept by the side of the body
- Hold for 10 seconds before returning to the front support and repeating on the other side
- Aim to keep the movement from one support to the other as controlled as possible

Progression: When in the side support position, slowly raise the upper arm and/or the leg. Keep the toes pointed, and the glutes and quads engaged.

Exercise 6.11 Back support (table top)

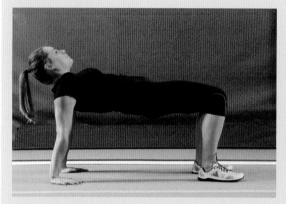

(a) Back support (table top)

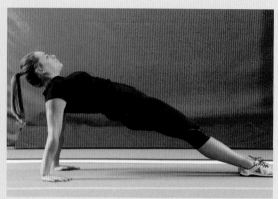

(b) Back support (straight legs)

The back support is often omitted in general fitness programmes, yet is a highly effective whole body-conditioning exercise that develops shoulder flexibility, and posterior chain strength and endurance that is transferable to a number of advanced skills.

Basic movement

- Sit on the ground with the hands placed shoulder width apart just behind the hips
- Bend the knees so the feet are flat, and push the hands and feet into the ground as you raise the body to a horizontal position (table top position)
- Hold this position for 10–30 secs, keeping the abdominals and glutes engaged, and the chin tucked throughout
- As you become stronger, begin the movement from a straight leg position
- Engage the abdominals, glutes and quads, and drive the hips and chest upwards to a fully extended back support position. Keep the arms straight, pushing them into the floor

Exercise 6.12 Super hero

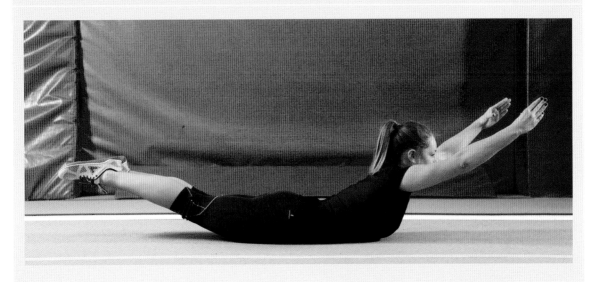

The super hero begins the process of extension patterning and offers a simple way to learn the correct body shape statically, before moving on to more dynamic variations. Training the extensor muscles as a group not only supports static postural control, but also the maintenance of upright postures during movement. The ability to move quickly from flexion to extension can also be useful in powerful movements such as the gymnastics round-off.

Basic movement
- Lie in a prone position with legs straight and elbows out to the side, resting your forehead on the back of your hands
- Engage the glutes and quads to stabilise the lower body
- Initiate extension by lifting the forehead and chest slightly off the floor and holding.

As you extend, imagine lengthening through the top of your head
- If this is challenging on the extensor muscles, push the forearms into the floor slightly to assist extension – visualise lifting the thoracic spine upwards
- As you become stronger and more aware of your extensor muscles, explore moving the forearms further out to the side, and then eventually overhead with arms fully extended

When you can hold the super hero position comfortably with the arms and legs on the floor, it's time to progress towards the super hero balance. If the double leg lift is too challenging, then the exercise can be regressed to lifting one leg at a time. In any case, focus on attaining the right shape before you increase the holding time.

Progression: see exercise 6.13, super hero rock

Exercise 6.13 Super hero rock

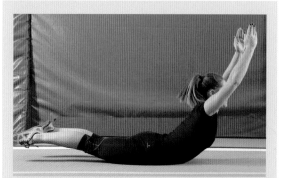

(a) Arms up

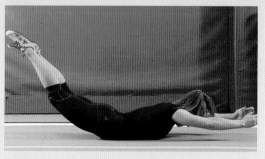

(b) Legs up

This progression challenges dynamic stability in extension.

- Assume the super hero balance position as before
- Begin a small rocking motion by quickly lifting the chest upwards – providing the body remains tight, this will cause the legs to roll down
- From here, allow the torso to roll back down under its own weight, reach forwards with the arms, and the legs will roll up
- Using this lifting and reaching action at the right points will maintain the rocking motion
- Build up your rocking time to 20 seconds

Exercise 6.14 Shoulder bridge

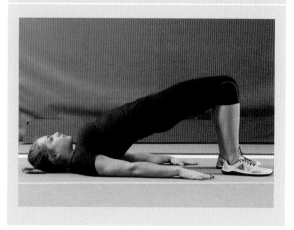

The shoulder bridge is a simple floor-based exercise that builds strength in hip extension, and serves as a stepping stone for advanced bridge progressions.

Basic movement

- Lie on your back with knees bent, feet flat on the floor; the ankles should be slightly in front of the knees, and the chin tucked in
- Keeping your arms by your side, engage the abdominals and glutes and drive the hips upwards until you form a straight line with the shoulders, hips and knees
- Hold for a few seconds before slowly returning under control

Exercise 6.15 Bridge press

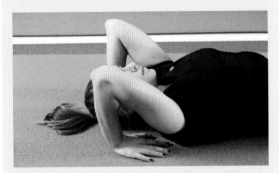

(a) Hand position

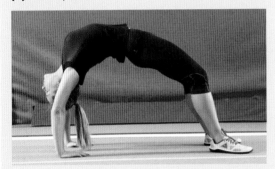

(b) Floor

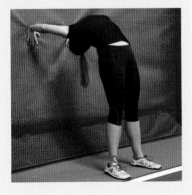

(c) Wall

The bridge press (also known as the bridge up or gymnastics bridge) is a challenging whole-body stability and strength exercise that requires a good level of shoulder flexibility in extension to perform skilfully and safely. However, for this reason it is a useful, yet advanced drill for skills that require shoulder stability in an open position, e.g. handstands.

Basic movement
- Lie flat on your back
- Bend your arms and put them flat on the ground by your ears, with forearms vertical to the floor
- Bend the knees and place your feet flat on the ground
- Engage the abdominals and glutes, and press through the shoulders and drive the hips up, raising the body off the floor
- Aim to straighten the legs as much as possible, pushing the head through your arms
- Although you may not reach anywhere near full arm or leg extension initially, a skilful bridge should finish with the arms vertical to the floor and the rest of the body in full extension

This exercise can be regressed to help individuals improve flexibility in shoulder and hip extension. The objective of the exercise is to focus on proper hip and shoulder extension. As you build flexibility and endurance, you can start to walk your hands further down the wall.
- Stand with your back facing a wall, about 2–3 feet away
- Keeping the feet a few inches apart, engage the abdominals and glutes, and lean backwards reaching the arms overhead to catch the wall behind you
- Aim to place your hands on the wall around shoulder height, keeping the arms as straight as possible

Developmental perspective

An important objective of natural motor development is control of the body against gravity. These antigravity movements firstly develop in the head and trunk, then at the hip, knee and ankle. Furthermore, antigravity movements must develop early on in both flexion and extension movements. Using these key developmental milestones as a model for developing bodyweight skills, it becomes apparent that the ability to stabilise in fundamental flexion/extension postures is an important pre-requisite not only for transitions between postures, but more importantly for the translation of those same postures into efficient locomotor and manipulative patterns.

DOUBLE AND SINGLE LEG STABILITY

Following a simple motor development model, lower-body stability is best developed in upright postures under the vertical force of gravity, using both double and single leg exercises. Following similar progressions to floor supports, the goal should initially focus on correct muscle-activation patterns that result in a specific body shape, before progressing on to dynamic exercises.

Double and single leg stability is essential to almost every human locomotor and manipulative skill, and is integral to many bodyweight disciplines, including gymnastics, dance and martial arts. Lower-body static exercises can build high levels of hip, knee and ankle joint stability vital for daily function and overall health; dynamic stability exercises such as squatting and lunging are highly dependent on static stability. To maximise proprioceptive feedback from the ground, the following exercises should be performed in bare feet, where possible.

Exercise 6.16 Scales

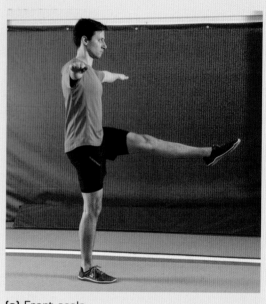

(a) Front scale

The standing scales are fundamental gymnastics drills that build correct muscle-activation patterns and help to control body shape and tension during more complex movements.

Basic movement
Front scale
- Stand with the feet together and engage the abdominals, glutes and quads
- Take the arms out to the side and roll the shoulders back to open up the chest
- Keeping both legs straight, slowly raise one leg out in front as far as comfortably possible, and hold for 10 seconds
- Repeat on the other leg
- Progress by increasing the height of the leg and hold for 30 seconds

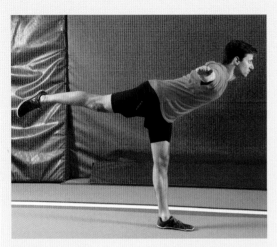

(b) Back scale

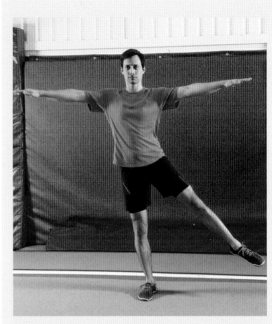

(c) Side scale

A dynamic progression of this exercise is front scale leg lifts.

- Assume the same set up position, and instead kick the leg up fast, and return slowly
- The toes should just lightly tap the floor, before immediately kicking the leg up again

Back scale

- Stand with the feet together and engage the abdominals, glutes and quads
- Take the arms out to the side and roll the shoulders back to open up the chest
- Keeping both legs straight and the torso tight, slowly lean forwards while simultaneously allowing one leg to raise behind you
- The rear leg should remain in line with the torso at all times, and the support leg should remain tight
- Hold for 10 seconds, repeat on the other leg
- Progress by increasing the height of the rear leg (and leaning further forwards), and increasing the holding time to 30 seconds

- A useful variation that further challenges balance and strength is to have the arms raised overhead during the hold

Side scale

- Stand with the feet together and engage the abdominals, glutes and quads
- Take the arms out to the side and roll the shoulders back to open up the chest
- Keeping both legs straight, slowly raise one leg out to the side as far as comfortably possible and hold for 10 seconds
- Repeat on the other leg

This exercise can be progressed by increasing the height of the leg and hold time to 30 seconds. The arms may also be raised to the overhead position to further challenge balance.

Exercise 6.17 Deep squat

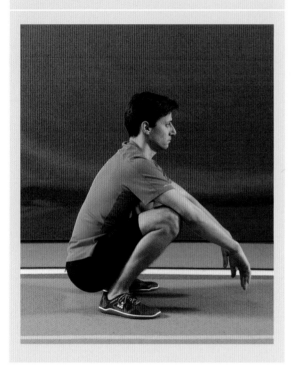

The deep squat, also known as the hunter-gatherer squat, is one of the most recognised and valuable bodyweight skills, as well as an important developmental milestone. The ability to deep squat with balance and control indicates optimal flexibility and structural balance between the hamstrings and quads. Deep squatting also improves mobility in the ankle, knee, hip and spine, and is an important prerequisite skill for efficient walking, running and lifting.

Basic movement

In standing, allow the feet to remain a natural distance apart – usually somewhere between hip and shoulder width. The feet should also be allowed to angle out to a natural 10–20 degrees.

- From this position, drop down as far as you can comfortably go into the deep squat position keeping your balance
- Keep the feet flat on the floor and ensure that pressure is directed towards the balls of the feet. The big toes should be rooted throughout. The arms may be held straight out in front of the body for balance
- Hold this position for up to 30 seconds, then drive the hips upwards and forwards to return to standing
- If your flexibility prevents you from achieving a balanced deep squat position, perform a partial range of motion squat; alternatively, perform the squat about 6 inches in front of a wall, and as you drop into the lowest position, lean your low back/pelvis into the wall for support
- Gradually increase the range as flexibility improves. Instead of holds, you can also perform the squat for repetitions

It's important to be patient and take things slowly, as the deep squat stretches muscles and tendons in a different way to the traditional parallel squat.

Progression: see exercise 6.18, single leg squat (bent knee)

Exercise 6.18 Single leg squat (bent knee)

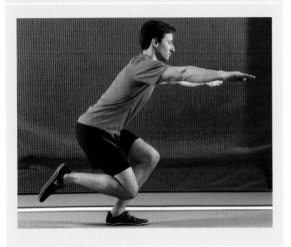

- From the start position, bend one knee to 90° and hold this position as you squat down on the other leg.

This position will allow you to squat further, but also requires more strength and balance. A further balance challenge can be added by holding the ankle of the bent knee, and reaching the free arm forwards as you squat.

What does the research say?

Opponents of the deep squat often cite protection of the knee as a major reason to avoid deep squatting. And it is often suggested that aside from few elite sports, the majority of activities don't require full knee flexion – making deep squats contradictory to specificity of training.

Indeed, early studies that looked at squatting and high knee-flexion angles suggested that there was an increase in collateral and anterior cruciate ligament laxity in Olympic lifters who regularly performed deep squats (Klein, 1961). The results of this study consequently led to a widespread belief that squat performance should not go below parallel, one that is still in place today. Interestingly, later studies have refuted Klein's findings (Meyers, 1971; Steiner et al, 1986; Chandler et al, 1989; Panariello et al, 1994).

When looking at the research as a whole, studies have demonstrated that the risk of injury to the knee is significantly lower in the deepest part of the squat. Anterior and posterior cruciate ligament forces have been demonstrated to diminish at high knee flexion angles (Markolf et al, 1996; Li et al, 2004; Sakane et al, 1997; Li et al, 1999). Deep squatting may also have a protective effect on the knee ligaments, due to compression of the soft tissue within the knee joint (Li et al, 2004) – in other words, there is reduced motion of the lower leg in the deepest part of the squat. While the greatest risk for injury during deep squatting would theoretically be to the menisci and cartilage, there is little evidence to show a cause-effect relationship in healthy subjects.

Finally, in terms of muscular development, deep squats can help to develop and maintain structural balance between the hamstrings and quads, increase glute activation more than parallel squats, and specifically target the vastus medialis obliquus muscle (Caterisano et al, 2002).

Exercise 6.19 Lunge

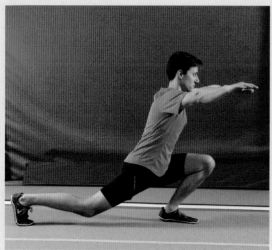

(a) Forward lunge

(b) Side lunge

Much like the squat, the lunge is a transitional movement; the only difference being that it develops our ability to handle loads when our feet are not symmetrical. Also, the lunge pattern has application to locomotion, for example running and jumping, where the jump takes off on a single leading leg during the run. Many tumbling skills in gymnastics also start with a lunge and reach, e.g. cartwheels.

Basic movement

- Stand with feet hip width apart, and step forward, bending the knee of the lead leg to 90°
- Allow the knee of the rear leg to bend, balancing on the ball of that foot
- Step out of the lunge by bringing the rear leg forwards back to standing
- Repeat for the desired repetitions before swapping legs

- Lunges can also be performed by stepping to each side, and may include reaching the arms overhead

SUSPENDED SUPPORTS

Suspended supports refer to body positions that involve the body being in a suspended position, usually from a high bar, chin-up bar, gymnastics rings, or similar. By nature, these positions rely solely on upper-body strength and endurance.

A few basic supports and levers will be explored in this section that once again build on the hollow body hold as a prerequisite. As these are advanced body positions, you are advised to focus on awareness of correct body shape, before you attempt to increase holding times.

Exercise 6.20 Front support suspended

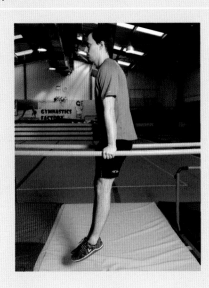

The upright front support is an essential exercise that will help maintain stability during exercises that require holding the body in an upright position with the legs suspended (e.g. rings, bar, wall, etc.). Dynamic control of this support can be found in advanced bodyweight exercises such as dips, muscle-ups and acrobatic movements such as vaults and flares. The exercise should preferably be performed using parallel bars or a dip machine, although the inside corner of a kitchen worktop or two sturdy stools may also be used.

Basic movement
- Lift yourself up onto the parallel bars and lock the arms out, as you support the body
- Engage the abdominals, glutes and quads, and assume a rigid, hollow shape

Progressions: see exercises 6.21, 6.22 and 6.23

Exercise 6.21 Front support rock

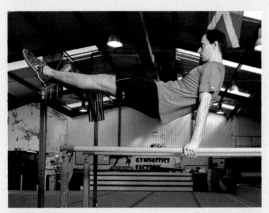

(a) Forward

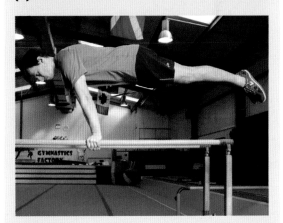

(b) Backward

- From the support position, gently rock forwards and backwards while maintaining a hollow shape and tight body
- The movement should be visualised as the torso rotating around a stable shoulder joint; focus on shape control rather than range of motion

Exercise 6.22 L-sit

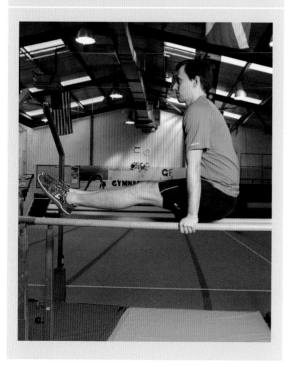

Exercise 6.23 Front support press

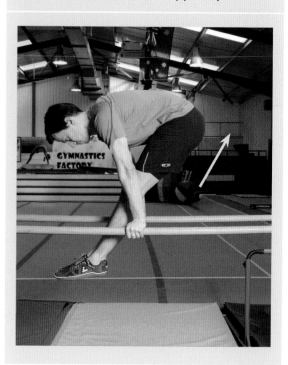

This exercise is best learned on the parallel bars, although it can be performed on the floor also. This is a challenging exercise, and use of the bars will allow you to hold the legs in a lower position until you develop the strength for the full L-sit (as well as reducing stress on the wrists).

- From the support position, maintain the hollow as you raise the legs to 90° hip flexion, holding for as long as you can with good shape
- As the legs rise, the hips will need to move behind the hands to maintain balance

This is a useful drill for learning the press to handstand, although it's also an excellent whole body-conditioning exercise.

- From the support position on the bars, press into the bars as you think about lifting the hips upwards
- In order to do this, you will need to hold a tight hollow shape throughout to maintain the axis of rotation

Exercise 6.24 Straight arm hang

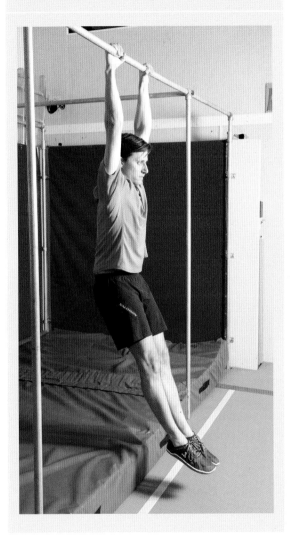

The straight arm hang is an important start position for a number of advanced dynamic bodyweight skills, such as swings, pull-ups, and muscle-ups. When performed with skill, this position will also build high levels of strength in the shoulder and core.

Basic movement

- Using an overhand grip, hang from a high bar with arms straight
- Assume the hollow shape, keeping the shoulders open, and the abdominals, glutes and quads engaged
- When performed correctly, the legs will hang forward of the torso
- Hold this position for 10–60 seconds

Progression: see exercise 6.25, straight arm swings

Exercise 6.25 Straight arm swings

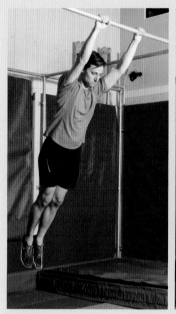
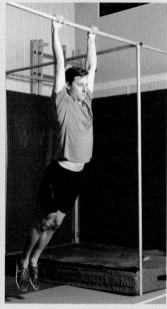
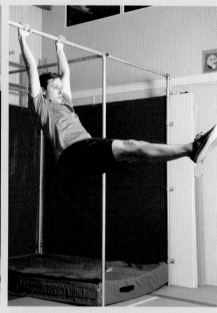

(a) Back swing (b) Extension (c) Forward swing

Once you are able to hold your body in the hanging position for at least 30 seconds, you can progress on to straight arm swings.

- Hang from the bar as before with the hands gripping as far over the bar as your forearm flexibility allows
- Keep the abdominals, glutes and quads tight, and initiate the swing by lifting the toes slightly forward
- Allow the legs to swing back (natural hip extension) and as your body moves back under the bar, quickly assume the hollow shape on the back swing
- To initiate the forward swing, release the hollow shape by extending the hips and opening the shoulders

- The abdominal/glute/quad tightness is essential to maintaining hip position under the bar and for a controlled swing, as opposed to an uncontrolled 'broken' sway

As swings become larger and more consistent, you may need to re-grasp the bar during the back-swing to maintain grip. A common mistake with swings is a loss of shape (and consequently momentum and control), as well as a tendency to pull with the arms, which can prematurely fatigue the biceps.

Exercise 6.26 Tuck front lever

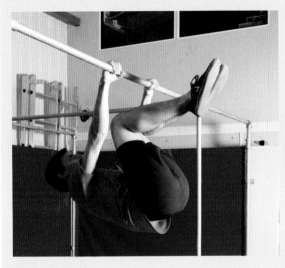

(a) Double leg

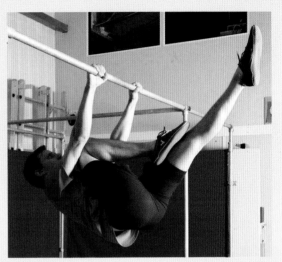

(b) Single leg

The front lever is an advanced movement that can be performed on a fixed bar or gymnastics rings. It's an impressive whole body, strength and endurance skill that can carry over into a number of other bodyweight skills and areas of performance. The exercise begins with the tuck front lever, before progressing to the fully extended front lever.

Basic movement

This exercise can also be performed on the rings.

- Begin in a hanging support position under a fixed bar, and engage the abdominals as you assume a hollow shape
- Keeping the arms straight, tuck the knees into the chest and lift the hips up towards the bar
- As the arms remain straight, the torso should rotate around the shoulder joints
- It's important to think about pulling the hands down towards the hips – this will help to engage the shoulder extensors
- In the full tuck front lever position, the hips should be at the same level as the head and shoulders, with the eyes looking straight up to the ceiling
- Note that in order to maintain balance, the shoulder joint will sit behind the wrist (when viewed from the side)

When you can hold the tuck position for 30 seconds, try extending a single leg for a hold.

- Begin with a small movement of the knee away from the chest, eventually reaching a straight leg position

This is a highly advanced skill, and it's important to spend time on the above steps and build up the required endurance and strength.

Exercise 6.27 Tuck back lever

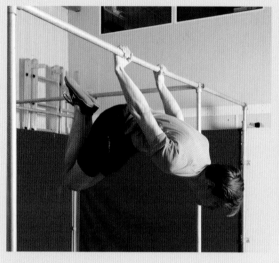

(a) Double leg

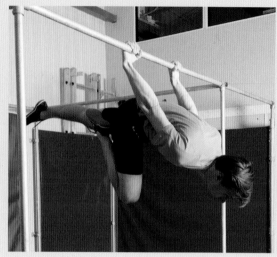

(b) Single leg

The back lever requires a high level of conditioning to achieve, and as such is an advanced exercise that requires a good foundation in bodyweight strength (namely dips, pull-ups and muscle-ups). As with the front lever, this exercise begins with a tuck back lever.

Basic movement
- Begin in a hanging support position under a fixed bar, and assume a tuck front lever position
- Continue to pass your knees up and over your head, and through your arms, until you are in a position where you are facing downwards ('skin the cat' position). Your arms will be rotated backwards and your shoulders will be under full stretch
- From this position, tuck the knees in to the chest and raise the hips to assume an upside down tuck position – head, shoulders and hips parallel to the ground

When you can hold the tuck position for 30 seconds, try extending a single leg for a hold.
- Begin with a small movement of the knee away from the chest, eventually reaching a straight leg position

HAND BALANCING
The following hand-balancing exercises will help to develop a strong foundation for, and efficiency in, a number of bodyweight skills. They will also serve to increase strength in the wrists, forearms and shoulders, providing a stable base of support for other ground-based bodyweight exercises.

Exercise 6.28 The crow

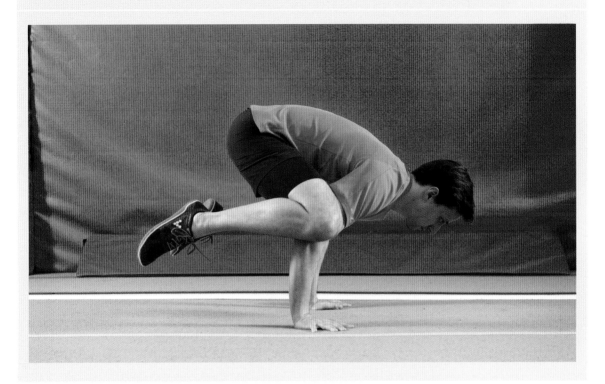

The crow is an excellent conditioning drill to help build endurance, stability and correct muscle-activation patterns for more complex skills, such as handstands.

Basic movement

- Kneel down on the floor and place the hands in front of the knees shoulder width apart, fingers pointing inwards slightly – this hand position will allow the elbows to bend slightly and flare outwards
- Come up on to the toes and place the knees on the outside of the arms, just above the elbows
- From here, gently rock forwards and backwards, transferring weight on to the hands, keeping the toes on the floor for support – this will help you find your balance point
- Repeat several times and rest
- Once you have a good feel for where your balance point is, lean forwards and slowly take one foot off the ground – the easiest way to do this is to point your toes
- Gently rock back and forth, switching from left to right foot
- Finally, lean forward and bring both feet off the ground, pointing the toes and squeezing the heels into the butt
- Aim to keep the hips low and look forwards as you hold this position.

Exercise 6.29 The crane

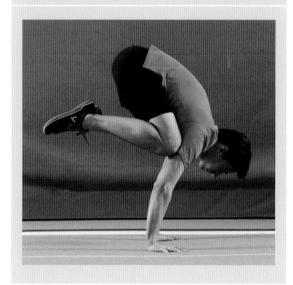

The crane is a progression of the crow that demands more strength, control and balance. The higher position of the hips will also start to train the body towards an inverted position.

Basic movement

- Kneel down on the floor and place the hands in front of the knees shoulder width apart, with the fingers pointing forwards. This hand position will allow you to rotate the elbow creases outwards to keep the arms locked out
- Come on to the toes and rest the knees on the back of the arms as close to the armpits as possible
- Note that having the knees in this position will raise the hips above shoulder height in this exercise
- As with the crow hold, gently rock back and forth to gain a sense of balance
- Initially, there may be some discomfort in the wrists, so ensure you don't over-balance – the wrists will strengthen up in time
- Repeat several times and rest
- To progress, rock back and forth, with an alternating leg lift. Finally, as with the crow hold, pick up both feet, point the toes and tuck the heels into the butt

Tripod exercises

Tripod progressions are a series of exercises that involve headstand movements, and are often used as part of progressions of the crow/crane holds, as well as for handstand training. The tripod can help get a sense of being upside down, while relatively stable. However, they are still challenging progressions, and should not be attempted by those with acute or chronic neck problems, or high blood pressure.

Headstand movements can be uncomfortable on the head, so it's recommended you use a rolled-up towel or small cushion under the head.

Tripod exercises will usually begin with the tripod hold. In this exercise, the hands are positioned as in the crane hold. The head is then placed in front of the hands, forming a triangle. The legs are straightened one at a time, and the feet are walked in towards the head and the butt is pushed upwards. From here (as with the crane) each knee is placed on the back of the upper arm as close to the armpit as possible. With both knees resting on the arms, this is the tripod hold.

The tripod extension progresses the tripod hold by extending the legs upwards – this can be challenging for the back extensors, so it's important to progress slowly with fewer reps. An advanced progression is the tripod pike extension, where the legs are extended straight up from the ground.

Exercise **6.30** Double arm lever

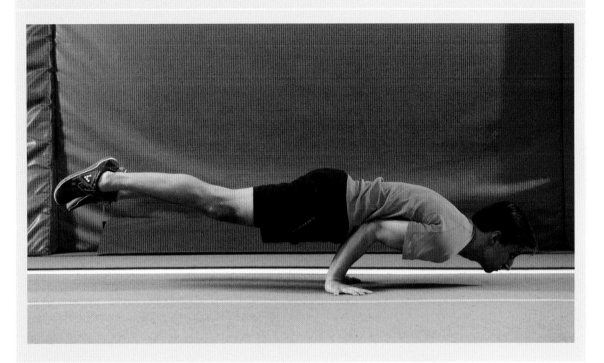

The double arm lever is not only a great whole body balance and strength exercise, it also forms part of the planche progression – a gymnastic skill in which the body is held parallel to the ground.

Basic movement
- From a kneeling position, place the hands on the ground in front of the knees (6 inches apart) with the fingers turned completely around so they are facing the knees. If this feels uncomfortable or you have limited flexibility in the forearm muscles to do this, turn the fingers out to the sides instead
- From here, bend the elbows and rest them against your stomach – this may feel uncomfortable at first
- Allow the head to rest on the floor somewhere in front of the knees
- From here, extend the knees so the legs are straight, toes touching the floor; at the other end, the head should still be lightly resting on the floor
- Hold this position while breathing naturally
- To progress to the full double arm lever, from the fully extended position above, lift the head off the ground first, followed by both legs, extending the body in a straight line from head to toe
- Engage the abdominals, glutes and quads to maintain this shape

Exercise 6.31 Handstand

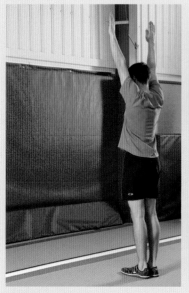
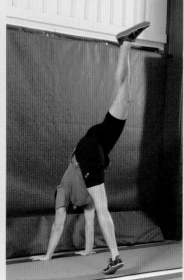
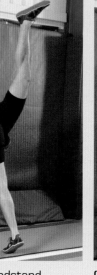
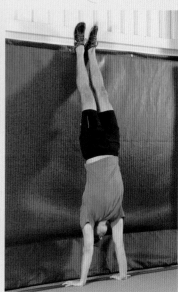

(a) Start position   (b) Kick up to handstand   (c) Handstand against wall

The handstand is one of the most visually impressive bodyweight skills, yet will take time to master the required strength, balance and coordination. While many different approaches exist to develop good technique, often the simplest is the most effective. With this in mind, it's important to drill basic pushing exercises such as push-ups and inverted presses, as well as static balance exercises such as the hollow hold, crow hold and crane hold. Once you have a good grounding in these movements, you can begin the following handstand progressions.

Basic movement

The outward facing wall handstand is probably the most common starting point for those ready to move on to the full handstand.

- Facing a wall, place the hands on the ground about six inches away from the wall and gently kick up to handstand with the feet coming to rest on the wall
- When in position, work at keeping the body straight with the head neutral; if the hands are too far away from the wall, there will be a tendency to arch the back or bend forwards
- Point the toes and visualise extending the body from the head through to the heels. Hold for no more than 10 seconds and gently return to standing

Progressions: see exercises 6.32, 6.33 and 6.34

Exercise 6.32 Lifting feet away from the wall

This progression will help you develop a feel for an unsupported handstand – and should you lose balance in this position, you can either fall back on to the wall, or kick down to standing.

- From the above position, lift one foot away from the wall maintaining a tight body shape
- Hold for a few seconds, return, and swap feet
- Alternate feet for 20–30 seconds and rest
- When you feel ready, try lifting both feet away from the wall and balancing for a few seconds

Exercise 6.33 Wall-facing handstand

This progression is psychologically more challenging as you will now require a safe exit strategy should you lose forward balance. The simplest exit strategy is to side-step out, e.g. if you feel like you're falling forwards, walk one hand towards the other hand and side-step down with the opposite leg.

- Stand with your back against the wall and walk your feet up the wall until you are in the handstand position. Your hands should be a few inches away from the wall
- Maintain a good shape and progress to lifting one foot away from the wall at a time
- When ready, try lifting both feet away

Exercise 6.33 Wall-facing handstand

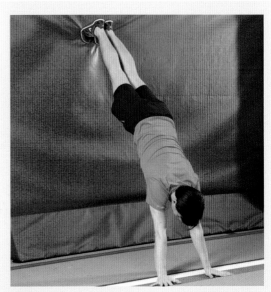

(a)

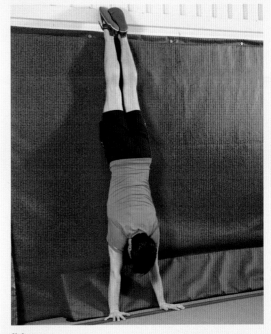

(b)

Exercise 6.34 Handstand (unsupported)

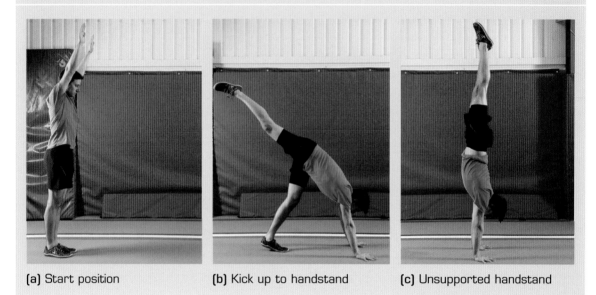

(a) Start position   (b) Kick up to handstand   (c) Unsupported handstand

Now that you know what it's like to balance momentarily in a handstand, and you have an exit strategy, it's time to progress to the unsupported handstand. Find a suitable space, and practise kicking up to balance. Remember to keep the body straight, and toes pointed.

Handstand tips

Use the following tips to make your handstand more efficient:

- Lunge long into the handstand. As a guide, your hands should be planted approximately one body length in front of you
- When planting the hands, spread the fingers with middle fingers pointing forward
- Push the hands into the floor as you kick up
- Keep both arms and back leg straight as you kick up
- Drive the hips over the shoulders during kick up – the quicker your hips are over your shoulders, the more balance you'll have

- Maintenance of body tension is the key to good balance and aesthetics; loss of tension often results in a banana-shaped handstand. The hollow-body hold is an essential exercise to master when perfecting the handstand, see page 69
- When practising unsupported handstands, use a partner to catch your legs as you kick up. They can then use small adjustments of your legs to fine tune your balance, while you focus on other aspects of the skill

Allow time between handstand sessions for the wrists to recover.

MANIPULATIVE SKILLS

7

INTRODUCTION

In human motor development, manipulative skills include pushing, pulling, lifting, striking, throwing, kicking and catching. While all of these are useful skills in adults, pushing and pulling are key patterns to develop further because of their transferability to other bodyweight skills. With this in mind, the focus of this chapter will be on these patterns.

Pushing is classified as a manipulative skill involving use of the hands. The skill of pushing bodyweight both horizontally and vertically takes place relatively early on, and is also a common movement found in adult daily life. Bodyweight pushing movements can therefore offer a simple way to enhance this skill and improve fitness for general health or sports performance.

In simple terms, bodyweight can be pushed away from a fixed point in three ways:
1. Horizontally, e.g. push-up
2. Vertically (arms overhead), e.g. inverted press
3. Vertically (arms down), e.g. dips.

These variations and their progressions will be explored in this section. To ensure adequate preparation for these movements, a warm-up that includes hollowing and front support drills

The importance of body shape during pushing movements

The term body shape refers to a particular body alignment during movement. For proper execution of many bodyweight exercises, the use of a hollow body shape is required, and allows the individual to stabilise the upper body with respect to the lower body, therefore ensuring that force production and transfer between upper and lower extremities is efficient during movement.

When drilling pushing movements, it is useful to adopt the hollow shape (see page 69 to learn the hollow shape) as it can transfer across to a number of advanced bodyweight movements.

is recommended to develop correct body shape. For details on how to perform the hollow body hold and front support, please refer to page 69.

Pulling is another important manipulative skill that usually develops from the age of 6 months onwards. In young children, its objective is to pull the body towards an upright position, e.g. pulling to a kneeling or standing position, as well as pulling objects towards the body. In adults, pulling is commonly combined with other manipulative skills such as lifting, however, certain recreational activities and sports may require significant amounts of stability, strength and coordination in pulling, and as such it's worth mastering basic pulls.

Bodyweight pulling movements are best drilled using a high bar or gymnastic rings, although most can be adapted using a simple pull-up bar, a suspension training system, and in some cases the edge of a sturdy table.

Bodyweight can be pulled away from a fixed point in two ways:

1. Horizontally, e.g. horizontal rows
2. Vertically (arms overhead), e.g. pull-up.

A third type of pull with the arms by the sides (inverted position) also exists, although as a bodyweight skill, this is rarely seen outside of gymnastics rings training. Therefore, this section will focus on the above two variations and their progressions. To ensure adequate preparation for these movements, a warm-up that includes hollowing and hanging support drills is recommended to develop correct body shape. For details on how to perform these drills, please refer to chapter 6 on Stability skills.

A foundation for pulling efficiency

While humans have evolved as bipedal specialists, other primate species remain climbing specialists, and show poor efficiency in walking. That is not to say that humans shouldn't climb – in fact, climbing movements are seen in a number of human activities from simple playing through to sport.

Climbing is a locomotor skill that employs pulling movements but is not exclusive to pulling. When performed with skill, climbing involves the legs as much (if not more, in some cases) as the upper body. Whether you are climbing rope, a wall, or a tree, the most efficient way is to maximise use of the legs and arms together. Even in cases, where the lower body is suspended, the most efficient way to get your body over your hands into a support position is to forcefully kick the legs, drive the hips towards the hands, and rapidly rotate the upper body forward – sometimes referred to as kipping.

So does this make the pull-up a redundant skill for humans? Quite possibly, and to answer this with another question – when did you last see a climbing specialist such as an chimpanzee do a pull-up? As previously discussed, from a point of locomotive efficiency, pulling should be optimised with the appropriate leg movements, and this is what other climbing specialists do well. However, what is often understated is that these specialists also exhibit another locomotive pattern that is essential for skilful pulling – brachiation or swinging. Swinging from bars and tree branches is a play activity in human children nowadays. However, it can be an effective foundational skill for efficient pulling. Other than a good grip, efficient hanging requires open shoulders and straight arms, and during swinging, it's essential that this position is maintained; any pulling with the biceps can cause early-onset fatigue. Hanging and swinging drills can build huge amounts of static and dynamic stability at the shoulder joint – which results in a stronger base for pulling movements, less stress on other joints, and better force transfer through the movement.

PUSHING MOVEMENTS

Exercise 7.1 Push-up

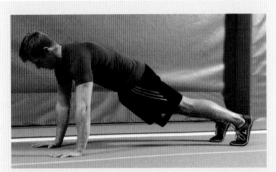

(a) Start

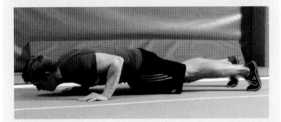

(b) Finish

Exercise 7.2 Long lever push-up

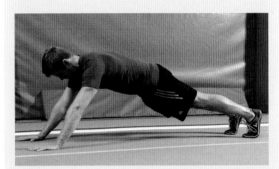

(a) Start

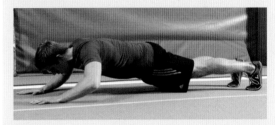

(b) Finish

Basic movement

- Assume a front support position, engaging the abdominals, glutes and quads; keep the hips open
- Maintaining this body shape and tension, bend the elbows and slowly lower the body towards the floor
- Pause momentarily before returning to the start position
- The exercise can be made easier by resting the lower body on the knees, instead of the toes, and moving the knees further away from the body as you become stronger

Progressions: see exercises 7.2–7.8

- Walk out the arms towards an overhead position, i.e. in front of the head
- This will significantly increase the amount of body tension required to hold the hollow shape, so take care not to over-reach initially
- Over-reaching can also cause the hands to slide away, however maintenance of a good hollow shape will minimise this

Exercise 7.3 Planche-lean push-up

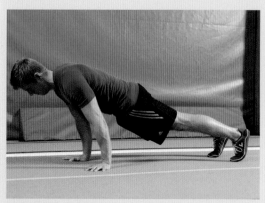

(a) Start

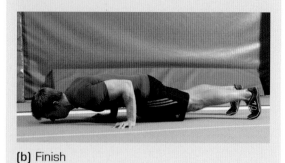

(b) Finish

Exercise 7.4 Wide hand push-up

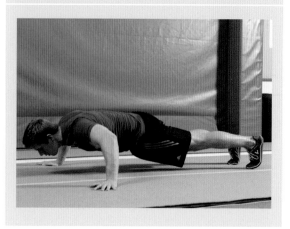

- Assume a push-up position as before, but place the hands out wide
- Perform the push-up, and repeat as necessary
- To challenge stability, take the feet out wide too

This progression dramatically increases the load at the shoulder joint and wrist, as well as introducing a balance component.

- Move the hands closer to the trunk, leaning the body forwards over the shoulders
- The hollow shape should be maintained throughout

Variations

Push-up variations can provide diversity of movement that is useful when building up to movement combinations and sequences, as well as being great conditioning tools.

Exercise 7.5 Staggered hands

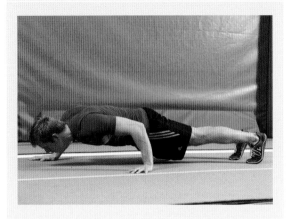

- Alternate one hand forward and the other one back to create further challenges to both trunk stability and the load through the shoulders, chest and arms

Exercise 7.6 Push-up with twist

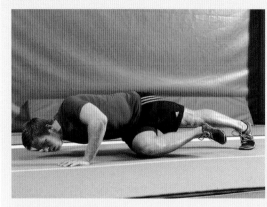

(a) Internal rotation

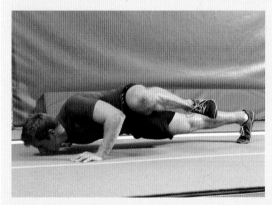

(b) External rotation

- Bring one knee towards the opposite shoulder as you lower the body (internal hip rotation)
- The knee may also be taken away from the opposite shoulder (external hip rotation)

Exercise 7.7 Archer push-up

Exercise 7.8 Explosive push-up

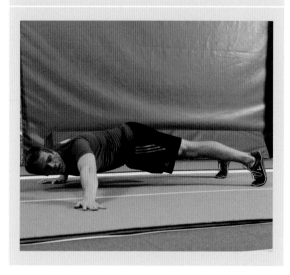

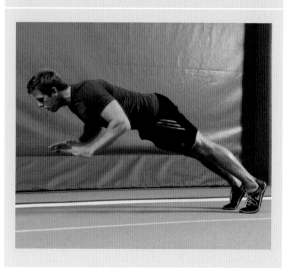

This variation requires both strength and coordination as a significant amount of bodyweight is alternated through each arm.

- From a wide hand front support position, lean over to one shoulder as you lower the body to the ground
- The other arm remains as straight as possible providing balance and support to the movement
- Push back to the start and repeat on the other side

- In this variation, explode upwards as soon as the body reaches its lowest position
- When performed with optimal power, the hands can be clapped, or quickly pulled in towards the shoulders before catching the body once again on the floor
- Other variations include catching the body in a wide/narrow/staggered hand position

Exercise 7.9 Inverted press

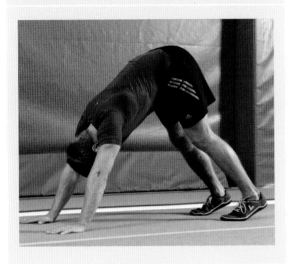

Exercise 7.10 Inverted press (legs elevated)

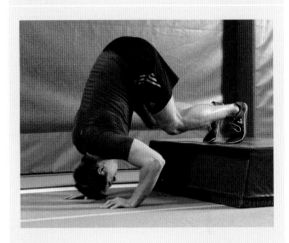

Basic movement

The inverted press progressively loads the upper chest, shoulders and triceps using a simple floor-based vertical push pattern. Note that this will be limited by hamstring flexibility, and a slightly bent knee position may need to be adopted.

- Assume the front support position, ready to perform a push-up
- While maintaining the hollow shape, walk the feet six inches towards the head, allowing the hips to lift upwards slightly
- The arms should still remain vertical (shoulders above wrists)
- From this position, lower the top of the head to the floor between your hands
- Return and repeat for the required reps
- As you become stronger, move the feet closer to the hands

Progressions: see exercises 7.10 and 7.11

- A progressive elevation of the legs will provide further challenges by increasing the load on the upper body

Exercise 7.11 Handstand push-up

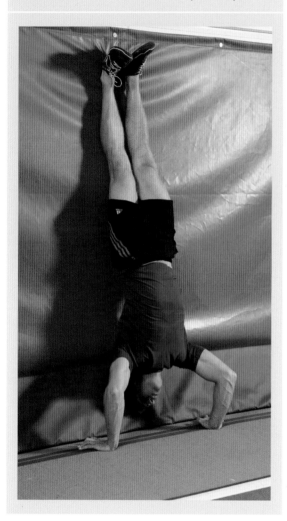

Continual elevation of the legs will eventually result in the handstand push-up. This is an advanced bodyweight exercise, and should not be attempted until you can perform a stable handstand against the wall. In any case, a wall should always be used for this exercise, and range of motion should be increased gradually. For more details on hand-balancing drills for handstand development, please refer to the section on stability skills.

- Begin by kicking up to handstand against the wall
- Assume a tight hollow shape and open the shoulders
- Bend the elbows as you lower the head towards the floor, only going as far as your strength allows
- Push back up to the start position

Exercise 7.12 Dips

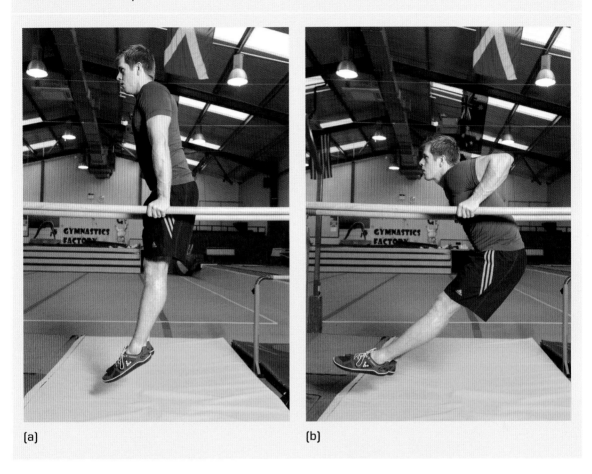

(a)

(b)

Basic movement

Dips require the use of parallel bars, a dip machine, or even gymnastics rings. The range of motion for this exercise will be limited by shoulder flexibility in extension; attempting to drop lower than your existing range may result in a loss of efficiency as the elbows flare out and the shoulders elevate to compensate.

- Place your hands on the bars and push down to lift your body to the upright suspended position

- Assume the hollow position and squeeze the arms into the sides pointing the elbow creases outwards
- Maintaining your shape, lower the chest to a point between your hands, push away, and return to the start position

Dips can be regressed by using an assisted dip machine, or via a partner/object supporting the legs.

PULLING MOVEMENTS

Exercise 7.13 Pull-up (with chin-up)

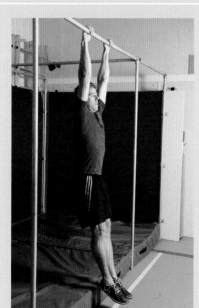

(a) Pull-up
(start)

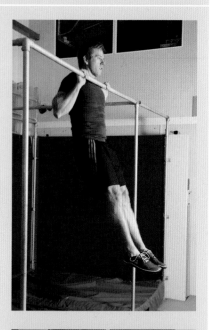

(b) Pull-up
(finish)

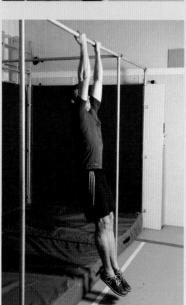

(c) Chin-up
(start)

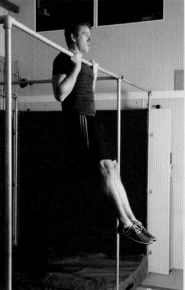

(d) Chin-up
(finish)

Basic movement

- Grab the bar with an overhand grip and assume the hollow shape position with abdominals, glutes and quads engaged
- Keeping the elbows close to the sides, pull the chest to the bar, and lower back to a fully extended shoulder position
- Keep the hollow shape throughout the movement. The exercise may also be performed with an underhand grip (known as a chin-up)

The pull-up and chin-up can be made easier by assisting bodyweight via an assisted pull-up machine, having a partner support the feet, or using a high resistance exercise band looped around the feet and anchored to the bar.

Progressions: see exercises 7.14–7.17

Exercise 7.14 Pull-up (rings)

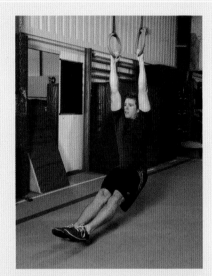

(a) Start

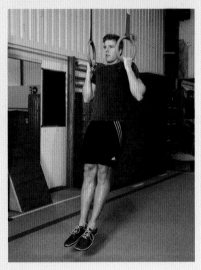

(b) Finish

Performing pull-ups on gymnastics rings offers a highly unstable anchor point, which significantly increases muscle activation throughout the upper body in an attempt to keep the movement controlled.

Exercise 7.15 Rotating pull-up

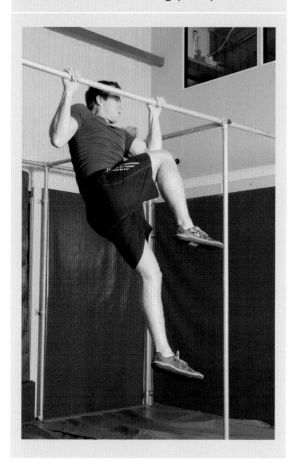

Exercise 7.16 Archer pull-up

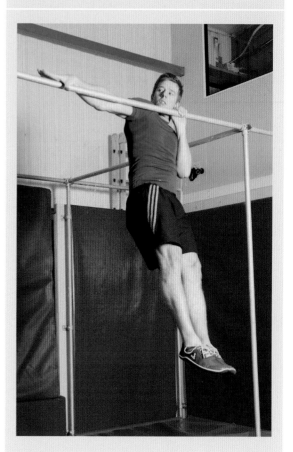

The aim of this exercise is to rotate the trunk and hips while performing a pull-up.

- Starting with the legs apart, perform a pull-up, while simultaneously rotating the trunk and bringing one knee to the opposite elbow
- De-rotate on the way down and immediately repeat with the other leg

As with the archer push-up, this variation alternates the pulling load from one arm to the other.

- From a full hanging position on the bar, assume a hollow shape
- As you begin to pull up, pull harder on one arm so that the body is pulled towards and underneath one hand; the other arm should move into a straight-arm position (like an archer pulling on a bow)
- Slowly return and repeat on the other side

Exercise 7.17 Kipping pull-up

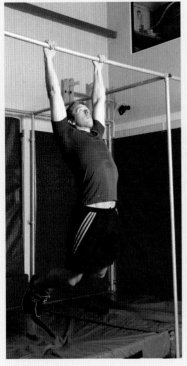

(a) Swing

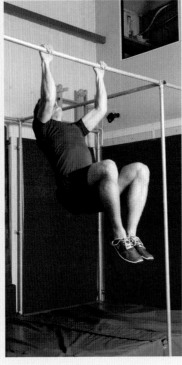

(b) Hollow and flex

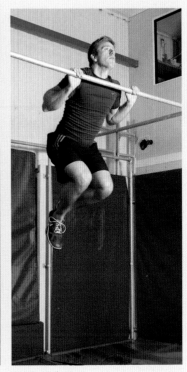

(c) Pull to bar

This is an excellent (advanced) conditioning exercise, as well as a preparatory drill for the muscle-up. Prerequisites for this movement include pull-up speed, as well as the ability to perform the straight-arm swings on a high bar.

- Grab the bar with an overhand grip and begin the swings (as previously described)
- As you move into the hollow shape on the back swing, immediately kick the toes forwards and simultaneously flex the knees and hips to 90°, pulling your body to the bar

- The transition from the arch to hollow combined with the explosive hip flexion will allow the body to be pulled to the bar efficiently
- Drop back down under the bar into the hollow shape

As you become stronger, you will be able to perform the movement without flexing the hip and knees.

Exercise 7.18 Horizontal row

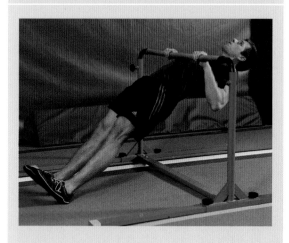

Basic movement

This exercise requires a fixed bar that is about waist height.

- Grab the bar, and suspend your body underneath, arms vertical and legs straight in front of the bar
- Assume a hollow shape and engage the abdominals, glutes and quads
- Maintaining this shape, pull your chest towards the bar, return and repeat
- The legs can be elevated to increase the load through the pull

The grip debate

The decision on which type of grip to use during pull-ups – wide, narrow, overhand, or under-hand is often debated. From an anatomical perspective, the overhand grip puts the forearm in pronation and places the shoulder at a mechanical disadvantage – forcing the latissimus dorsi to work more. Therefore, from a training standpoint, wide or narrow doesn't really matter, and it's more a question of overhand vs. under-hand grip.

It's also important to consider that any limitations in shoulder motion – whether this is from injury or lack of flexibility – may be best addressed with a change in grip to one that suits the individual's current functional ability. In this way, a training effect can still be gained without unnecessary risk of (re) injury.

What's interesting to note is that in a natural environment, the overhand pull-up is the movement of choice, especially when the pull-up is used as the first step in pulling the body up and over the hands (i.e. muscle-up). In addition, maintaining a narrow grip will be more efficient, especially if the pull-up is combined with a kipping movement. With this in mind, those involved in outdoor activities such as climbing or Parkour may prefer to train predominantly with an overhand narrower grip.

LOCOMOTOR SKILLS

INTRODUCTION

Locomotor skills are traditionally classified as motor skills that use the feet to move the body from one place to another, and in humans, include walking, running, hopping, jumping, skipping, galloping, sliding, and leaping. There are three functional features of any locomotor pattern:

1. Stability
2. Propulsion
3. Efficiency.

While locomotor skills are learned and developed progressively in childhood, adults can adapt and practise many of these fundamental patterns to improve fitness for daily life and sport. Moving from one place to another can also involve arms as well as legs, and your locomotor skills can expand to quadrupedal motor patterns (many of which are based on primitive patterns of creeping and crawling) and even tumbling movements.

This section explores the patterns of walking, running, jumping, vaulting, quadrupedal patterns, sweeps and basic tumbling, and how they can be progressed and varied as part of a bodyweight training programme. Later chapters will explore ideas for integrating these patterns into more complex movement skills and sequences.

WALKING

Walking is the most common form of human locomotion, and when performed with good mechanics is an extremely efficient movement pattern. Walking is defined by a pendulum action in which the body essentially moves over the stable limb with each step. During walking, only one foot at a time loses contact with the ground, and there is always a period of double support (when both feet are on the ground). This results in a very stable movement that has a loading force of approximately 1 x bodyweight, with a long contact time on the ground. Walking is regarded by many biomechanics experts as the 'first gear' of natural human locomotion.

While we often assume we can walk reasonably well, our abilities to maximise efficiency are often clouded by reduced proprioceptive feedback from the ground – we've lost our sense of our feet meeting the ground – especially because we're used to wearing shoes. A significant proportion of proprioceptive feedback to our nervous system comes from our lower half, and it is believed that a large chunk of this comes from the sole of the foot (plantar surface). If this feedback gets filtered out, for example through use of inappropriate footwear, then so does our feedback. As a result, we begin to make inappropriate shapes with our body, which can result in loss of efficiency, impaired movement and potential injury.

While it's not the intention of this text to explore the mechanics of walking in any depth, it's important to understand proper walking mechanics as the foundation of running, sprinting and other locomotor patterns. Here are a few considerations to be mindful of, not only during your training, but in everyday activities also.

1. **Go barefoot** – as soon as you take your shoes off, you will immediately start maximising proprioceptive feedback. The more time you spend with bare feet, the quicker your body will learn to adapt by making full use of the foot and ankle. Where permitted, do your bodyweight training with bare feet or wearing appropriate barefoot shoes.

2. **The 3 rockers** – during walking, the foot/ankle uses a 3-rocker mechanism: the heel rocker (heel strike); the ankle rocker (body moves over foot); and the forefoot rocker (heel lifts). Being mindful of this during walking will improve feedback and efficiency of movement.

3. **Axis of leverage** – during walking, the human foot transmits weight from the heel, along the outside of the foot, across the ball of the foot and finally through the big toe. Therefore the big toe is important for both balance and force production. As well as being mindful of this force distribution during walking (i.e. pushing off through the big toe) regular practice of foot and ankle mobility exercises (pages 33–38) will help to strengthen and mobilise the big toe.

RUNNING

If walking is the first gear of natural human locomotion, then running is the second. The switch to a running pattern is speed-dependent – as walking speed increases, there will be a point when the body will naturally change shape (posture) to one that is efficient for running. This is characterised by both feet being off the ground with each step (flight). This flight phase creates a larger impact force with foot strike, (approximately 2 x bodyweight with each strike). It's important to understand that in a natural habitat (i.e. barefoot), the most appropriate and efficient shape for the body is to remain upright and adopt a forefoot strike with a momentary heel stroke.

Unfortunately, footwear with padded soles/heels not only filters out the feedback from ground contact, but also allows for a heel strike. Research has shown than heel strikers are more likely to suffer from running-related injuries compared to those who forefoot strike (van Mechelen, 1992; Taunton et al, 2003; van Gent et al, 2007).

There are a number of useful resources to improving running technique, many of which advocate barefoot technique as an important prerequisite – please refer to the recommended reading list at the end of this book for more details. Here are a few considerations when integrating running technique into your bodyweight training programme:

1. **Posture** – a relaxed, upright posture is the most important factor for efficient running technique. The legs should move in a cyclical manner (as opposed to a shuffling or pendulum-like movement). Each foot strike should occur under the centre of gravity, landing on the ball of the foot (forefoot). Running in bare feet on

a treadmill will help to drill optimal posture and foot strike in a relatively safe environment. It's important to understand that correct posture will optimise foot strike and subsequent loading. When making the transition to a forefoot strike outdoors, it's advisable to wear appropriate barefoot shoes that are anatomically shaped, offer protection, and provide maximum sensory feedback from the ground.

2. **Cadence** – in order to maximise the body's elastic system (and therefore minimise muscular effort), cadence (number of steps per minute) will need to increase. Observational studies have shown that elite middle distance runners run at cadences of 170–190 bpm. Many recreational runners will often fall short of this range, running in the 150–160 bpm range with longer strides and ground contact times. While they may not want to run faster, taking shorter strides will allow them to hit a higher cadence, and make better use of the elastic properties of the foot and ankle.

3. **Overstriding** – overstriding occurs when the foot strike is in front of the body's centre of mass. This will apply a repetitive braking force to the body with each foot strike, and will often result in a forward head position, a bend at the hips, and a long trail leg – all of which results in poor economy of effort. Longer strides also mean longer contact times, less elastic recoil, more muscle action and consequently more fatigue.

4. **Leg pull** – the pull of the rear leg is important to running efficiency. Efficient runners will have no pause at the completion of the leg's follow-through – the leg pulls back rapidly and immediately the knee drives forward (the cyclical motion mentioned earlier). As running speed increases, the magnitude of the pull from the hamstrings should also increase allowing for a greater stride length. Forward propulsion is the result of these quick leg pulls and minimum contact times on the ground, as opposed to 'pushing' the ground away.

Theory into practice

While running may be considered the purest, most natural form of bodyweight training, it is still a skill, and as such should be drilled and practised appropriately and progressively. While there are a number of useful exercises and drills within this text that can be used to master efficient running technique as part of an integrated bodyweight training programme, they are by no means exhaustive. With this in mind, the reader is strongly advised to seek out suitable education that provides both a sound biomechanical basis for improving running technique, as well as hands-on practical experience.

SPRINTING

Sprinting is the third gear of natural human locomotion, and exhibits slightly different body shapes and associated forces, compared to walking and running. At maximal speed, there are significant loading forces, however this is over a very small contact time (less than 0.1 seconds) – characterised by a forefoot strike with an absence of a heel stroke. Although posture should still remain upright, the arms will cycle through a greater range of motion, and cadence will be well above 200 bpm in elite sprinters.

Practical applications of walking and running within a bodyweight training programme

Walking and running have long been used within cardiovascular training programmes, and are often performed for longer durations. However, they can be scaled down to play an important role within a bodyweight training programme.

If you're training outdoors then walking can be used as an effective active recovery between bouts of bodyweight exercises, e.g. going for a 30 second walk in between Tabata cycles. For added intensity, walk up (and down) a steep bank.

Running drills can be applied in a similar way, for example, as an active recovery, or even as an exercise drill in itself. Integrating short runs and sprints into an interval-based bodyweight programme can add a significant level of metabolic conditioning to even the most simple of bodyweight training programmes. On the other hand, running can be used as the prime conditioning tool with other bodyweight exercises added in along the way, e.g. running a trail, and stopping at various points to perform push-ups, pull-ups, squats etc.

If you do decide to incorporate walking, running and sprinting in your training, do this in bare feet where appropriate, to maximise proprioceptive feedback from the ground.

It's important to understand that as running speed increases so do the forces placed on the body, as well as the stabilisation demands. As such, sprinters need to be stronger – specific running-related bodyweight drills can go a long way in meeting this strength requirement.

JUMPING

Jumping is an excellent conditioning activity that can be done almost anywhere with minimal or no equipment. The inclusion of vertical and horizontal jumping drills within a training programme can help to develop high levels of power that can transfer to a number of other activities and various sports.

Jumping is the transfer of weight from one or both feet to both feet, or in the case of hopping, to the same foot. All forms of jump can be divided into three phases: take-off, flight and landing. All three phases can be optimised for efficiency,

however, landing safely is an important skill to focus on when first learning to jump, hop or leap. An important extension of jumping is vaulting – made popular in mainstream fitness by the Parkour and free-running community – the basics of which will also be discussed.

JUMPING PROGRESSIONS

Whether jumping activities are chosen to meet general fitness objectives, or those of sports performance, it's important to progress in the right way to minimise the risks inherent with jump training. The following sequence of drills focuses on key patterns of movement that will build jumping skill. It's important to master each step before moving on to the next, although each one can be progressed within its own right if required. At every stage, there should be a continual emphasis on good position, coordination and fluidity of movement.

Exercise 8.1 Plyometric bounces

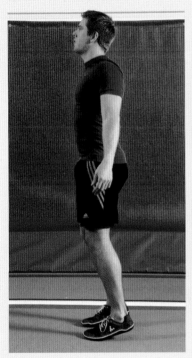
(a) Double leg

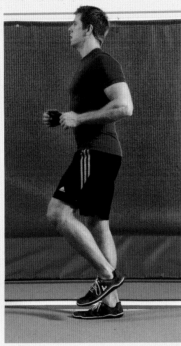
(b) Single leg

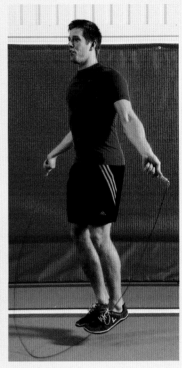
(c) Jump rope

These drills will help to develop the elastic potential in the foot and ankle, as well as teach quick ground reaction, and improve balance and posture. They serve as an excellent starting point for other progressions, as well as a warming up activity.

Basic movement

* In a standing position with feet no more than hip width apart, begin to bounce on the balls of your feet

* Aim for a rhythm of 180 bpm (use a metronome to assist you), and with each foot strike, the heel should 'kiss' the ground
* Hands, arms and shoulders should remain relaxed, and the focus should remain on bouncing on the same spot for 30–60 seconds

Progressions:

a. increasing time
b. hopping (single leg bouncing)
c. jumping rope

Exercise 8.2 Landing

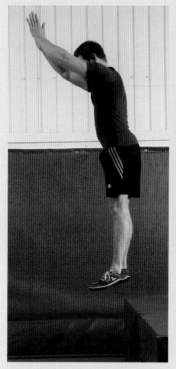

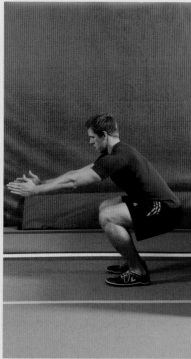

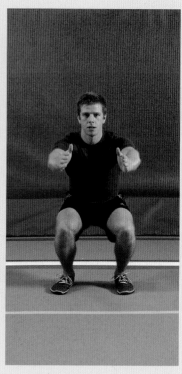

(a) Proper landing mechanics (jump)

(b) Proper landing mechanics (land)

(c) Proper landing mechanics (front view)

Efficient landing mechanics should be emphasised at the beginning of any jump training to include proper use of the ankle, knee and hip, as well as foot strike. At this stage, it's best to begin with a jump down from a small block or step. The effort should be gentle, with the aim of landing quietly on a full foot and sticking the landing. Adequate shock absorption will come from bending the ankle, knee and hip into a controlled 'collapse', and keeping the knees in line with the first and second toes on landing. Progressions may include increasing block height and increasing jump distance, as well as single leg lands.

Exercise 8.3 Squat jump

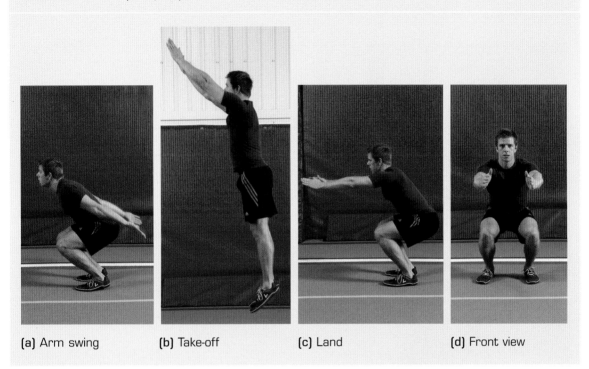

(a) Arm swing   (b) Take-off   (c) Land   (d) Front view

Once proper landing has been mastered on double and single legs, it's time to drill proper use of the arms during take-off. To keep things simple, this can be performed via a simple squat jump into the air.

Basic movement
- Begin standing with feet hip to shoulder width apart, hands by your sides
- Rapidly drop to a ½ squat position taking the arms behind the body. The moment you hit this bottom flexed position, forcefully swing the arms to transfer momentum to the whole body as you explosively extend the body and jump upwards

- Maintain a hollow body shape at the top of the movement, and aim to land with knees bent and aligned over the first/second toes, arms out in front for balance. It's important to keep the transition between the eccentric and concentric phases of the movement as short as possible – also known as the amortization or coupling phase – to maximise the elastic potential of the tendons and muscles

Progressions: tuck jumps or jumping onto a box (see exercise 8.4).

Exercise 8.4 Squat jump (jumping onto a box)

- Begin standing with feet hip to shoulder width apart, hands by your sides
- As with the basic squat jump, rapidly drop to a ½ squat position. The moment you hit this bottom flexed position, forcefully swing the arms forwards and upwards as you explosively extend the body and jump towards the box
- Land on the box with knees bent and aligned over the first/second toes

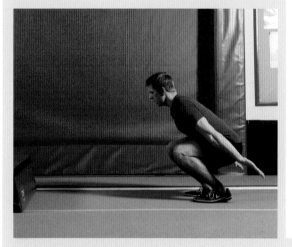

(a) Arm swing

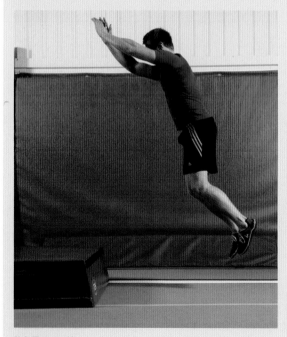

(b) Take-off

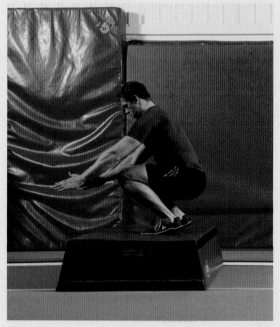

(c) Land

Exercise 8.5 Depth jumps

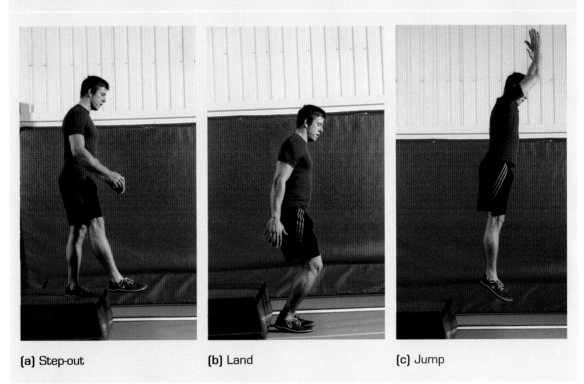

(a) Step-out   **(b)** Land   **(c)** Jump

These drills involve jumping down from a box and immediately jumping upwards/forwards. The nature of the movement allows for greater eccentric loading of the hips and legs, which potentially increases power output. Due to the higher demands placed on the nervous system, depth jumps require a solid training base and mastery of the first three steps. The key to an efficient depth jump lies in the ability to coordinate the step off and arm swing, as well as controlling the larger eccentric forces as you drop down.

Basic movement

- Begin by standing on a stable box or step that is 12–16 inches high
- Step out with one leg, with the aim of landing on both feet somewhere in front of the box – as you begin to step out, simultaneously swing the arms back
- Stick the landing with soft knees, allowing the ankles, knees and hips to bend further to absorb the force – by this point, your arms will have swung back fully
- Now, forcefully swing the arms forwards and explosively jump up
- Land once more, with proper foot strike, alignment, and shock absorption

Other jump progressions and variations

While the earlier progressions will provide a solid foundation for jump training, here are a couple of variations to try:

a. Jumping over an object (see exercise 8.6) – whether indoors or outdoors, objects may be used in jump training. These can be strategically placed and jumped over. In any case, practise double and single leg take-offs.

b. Precision jumps (see exercise 8.7) – a jump from a standing or running position on to an obstacle that often has a minimal surface area, such as a wall or a rail. The fundamental difference between a standing/running long jump and a precision jump is the level of skill required to 'stick' the jump on landing. In order to do this, the trajectory must be as accurate as possible to avoid over- or under-reaching, and ultimately falling off the obstacle.

Exercise 8.6 Jumping over an object

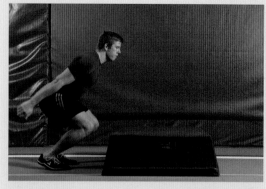

(a) Arm swing

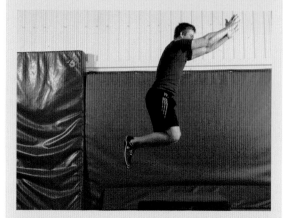

(b) Jump

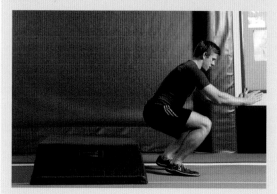

(c) Land

Exercise 8.7 Precision jump

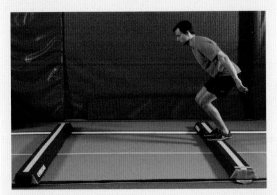

(a) Arm swing

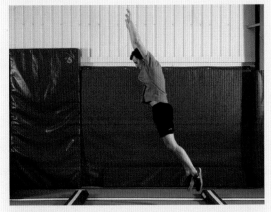

(b) Take-off

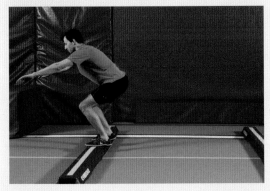

(c) Land

Theory into practice: jumping and trunk stability

The maintenance of trunk stability during jumping is essential to the overall efficiency of any particular jump. For example, consider a simple 2-legged standing jump. If there is poor stability through the trunk, there may be a tendency to over-extend or over-flex the trunk, resulting in unnecessary rotational forces. These will at best require stabilisation through additional muscular effort, and in the worst case, result in a loss of balance. Assuming a hollow body shape at take-off will ensure optimal midline stability that will not only provide a stable base for take off (and potentially better force transfer vertically), but also for landing.

Because jumping on the ground is a relatively quick action, we often don't have enough time to fully sense what it's like to have the correct (or incorrect) body shape at take-off. However, for those who have access to a gymnastics facility, using a trampoline can assist in bringing about better postural and positional awareness in a short space of time. Jumping on a trampoline allows for more airtime (greater height), resulting in a larger window for proprioceptive feedback. If body shape is less than optimal during this time, it will result in a noticeable rotation and loss of balance. You will quickly respond by making the right shape to attain better midline stability or not jumping as high.

It's also important to note that when it comes to landing, even a slight displacement of the feet in front of, or behind the body's centre of mass, will result in rotation and loss of balance; this balance awareness is extremely useful when transferring back to jumping on the ground.

VAULTING

While vaulting is a highly technical discipline in artistic gymnastics, the fundamental skill of vaulting is as useful to the bodyweight enthusiast, as it is fun and challenging. Vaulting is essentially a modified jump (with support) that allows the body to efficiently navigate obstacles generally deemed too high for jumping alone. Establishing a stable base of support (the arm and shoulder) that the rest of the body can move across, is vital for proper execution.

Few fitness facilities will have the required equipment to perform basic vaults, fortunately the outdoor environment will have plenty of options to practise the basic skills. It's important to look for a sturdy wall or railing that is mid-thigh to hip height, and is safe and large enough to place your hand on (or grip, in the case of a railing).

This section explores a few basic vault progressions which can be performed subsequently as standalone bodyweight conditioning drills, as well as being integrated into longer movement sequences.

Progressions for step vault

The following progressions begin with the basic step vault and build up to the speed vault – a vault popularised in Parkour and free running – which allows for efficient movement over an obstacle with minimal loss of momentum. The step vault progressions will also build a good foundation that can be transferred to other types of vaults.

This vault requires a stable box, low bar, or wall (about hip height). It's also worth noting that most right-handed people will prefer to place their left hand on the bar when vaulting, and jump their legs to the right. The progressions below are described for a right-handed individual, although the reverse should be practised for left-handed individuals, or to promote balance.

Exercise 8.8 Hand placement

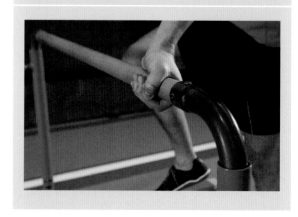

- Begin by standing behind the bar and placing your hand on the bar, as if about to vault over it
- An underhand grip (forward-facing palm) will encourage stability during the vault
- Practise walking up to the bar several times and placing the hand in this way

Exercise 8.9 Foot placement

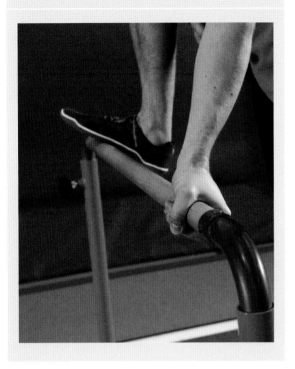

Exercise 8.10 Leg lift

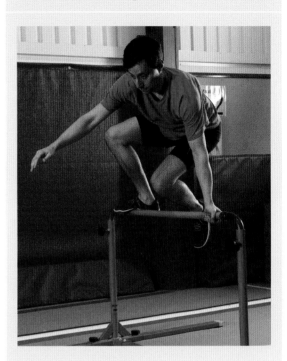

- As you walk up to the bar and place the hand, bring the right knee up and place the right foot on to the right side of the bar
- Aim to place the ball/mid-foot on the bar
- Repeat several times

- Walk up to the bar and place the hand and foot as previously described
- Apply downward pressure through the left arm and right leg so that you can support your bodyweight and lift the left leg off the ground
- You should be able to balance in this position comfortably with equal weight through the left arm and right leg
- Repeat this sequence several times

Exercise 8.11 Threading the leg

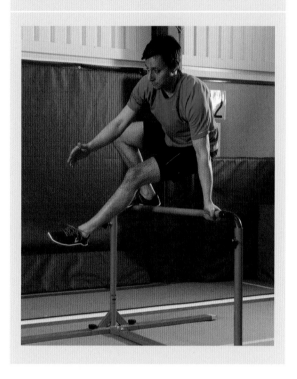

Exercise 8.12 Step out

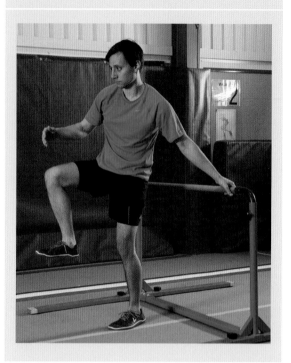

This next progression will help to build stability and control as the body moves over the bar.

- Walk up to the bar and place the hand and foot
- Lift the left leg and thread it through the body and sit down on the bar (maintaining the hand and foot placement)
- As the leg is threaded through, it's important to lean the chest slightly forwards to maintain balance and reduce effort
- Practise this several times

- Thread the left leg and fully extend the left hip as you step out on to this leg
- Release the right foot and left hand and walk away
- Repeat several times

Step vault

The full vault can now be performed by either walking or running up to the bar, and stepping through with control and fluidity. As speed increases, you can jump the right foot to the bar for added efficiency. Aim to maintain momentum by stepping out and continuing to walk/run, and keep the head facing forward throughout.

Exercise 8.13 Speed vault

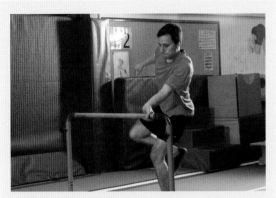

(a) Place hand

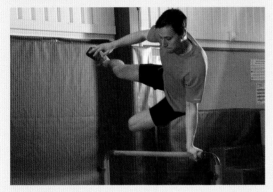

(b) Vault

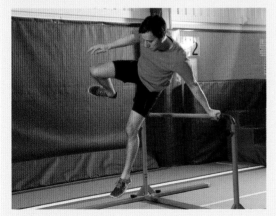

(c) Follow through

This progression of the step vault is useful when running towards an obstacle at faster speeds with the aim of maintaining speed out of the vault. The fundamental difference is that the speed vault does not place the right foot on the bar.

Basic movement

- As you run up to the bar, place the left hand, and swing the right leg over the bar, threading the left leg and stepping out
- By remaining balanced as you travel over the bar, you should be able to maintain forward movement without a loss of speed
- At higher running speeds, contact times can be further reduced by launching into the vault before the hand is placed on the bar
- In this progression, the right leg is swung out over the bar with the left threading through as normal
- As the body moves over the bar, the left hand is momentarily placed to maintain control and stability of the torso, and prevent excessive rotation

Exercise 8.14 Kong vault

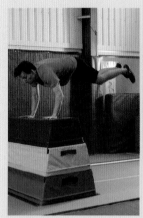
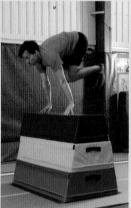
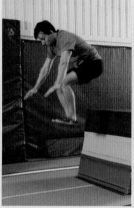
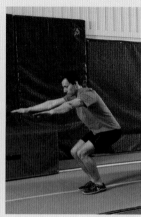

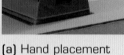
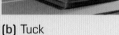
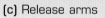

(a) Hand placement (b) Tuck (c) Release arms (d) Land

Popular in Parkour and free running, this vault variation brings both legs underneath the torso (and through the arms) landing on both feet.

Basic movement
- Stand in front of an object that has enough landing room on top of it
- Place your hands on the object and jump up landing on top of the object in a deep squat position
- As you jump, press the hands into the surface, engage the core and tuck the knees – as the feet are about to land, lift the arms up to rotate the body and land
- As you improve, start to lean forwards over the arms to generate forward momentum, aiming to land further forwards on the object
- It's important to release the hands from the surface before your feet land

- When you have drilled this several times, find a suitable obstacle that you can now practise vaulting over (e.g. wall, railing)
- Stand in front of the object and plant your hands on it. Push into the surface as you jump and tuck your legs through the arms
- Keep leaning forwards and as your knees pull through, release the arms and reach them out in front ready to balance you on landing
- Land on two feet in a balanced position
- As your confidence and technique grows, try clearing greater distances

QUADRUPEDAL PATTERNS

Quadrupedal movement patterns are one of the fastest growing bodyweight training trends, although their use has been widespread in physical therapy and mixed martial arts for many years. More recently, a number of fitness pioneers have developed mainstream training systems that incorporate quadrupedal exercises that have been influenced by human and 'animal' movement patterns, for example, Mike Fitch's Animal Flow, Scott Sonnon's BodyFlow, and Alvaro Romano's Ginastica Natural.

The interest in natural human and animal movements among fitness professionals has no doubt been a launch pad for the popularity of quadrupedal exercises; however, the rationale for their inclusion in fitness training is often misunderstood.

Following stability development during the first four months of life, there is a period that focuses on purposeful dynamic function of the arms and legs. During this time, locomotor function develops via two pathways: an ipsilateral or same-side pattern (turning) and a contralateral pattern or opposite side pattern (creeping and crawling). The ipsilateral pattern involves stepping the same side arm and leg forward (reaching) as the opposite side supports the body; the contralateral pattern develops on all fours where the opposite arm and leg step forward.

As well as being an important motor development milestone in humans, from a fitness perspective, quadrupedal patterns are dependent on good stabilisation to allow for efficient, purposeful movement. To optimise stabilisation, adequate mobility must also be established through some form of flexibility training. Quadrupedal patterns can be modified and progressed in adults to provide challenging whole body exercises that will appeal to any bodyweight enthusiast.

Several quadrupedal movement patterns are discussed below that can be used as simple drills in isolation, or when mastered, be effectively integrated into innovative bodyweight movement sequences.

Isolated vs. integrated stabilisation

If a client or athlete can contract and isolate muscle groups like the transversus abdominis or gluteus medius, it's no guarantee that these muscles will be used effectively during task-driven (functional) activities.

As well as being able to contract, stabiliser muscles must also use accurate timing and coordination to stabilise joints. The conscious contraction of these muscles does not occur in natural movement – it shouldn't require a lot of thought to activate the stabilisers, which should be under reflex control.

The use of quadrupedal crawling patterns (and other purposeful bodyweight movements) shifts the emphasis of the exercise away from muscle contraction, and towards completion of a task. This shift will in turn promote reflex stabilisation (without coaching or cueing), ultimately resulting in better movement in the extremity joints.

Exercise 8.15 Prone crawl

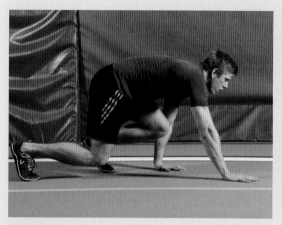

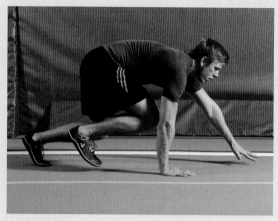

(a) 4-point

(b) 2-point

The prone crawl pattern is a good place to start if you are new to quadrupedal patterns. From here, a number of variations/progressions will be explored that will further challenge your bodyweight training.

Basic movement

- Begin in a 4-point kneeling position with the arms and knees positioned vertically under the shoulders and hips respectively
- Lift the knees a few inches off the ground – readjust your hand/foot placement (if needed) to maintain a balanced position
- Begin to lean forwards, as you reach the right hand and place it on the floor about 6 inches in front; immediately step forwards with the left foot to reposition your centre of mass over your hands/feet

- Repeat on the other side and continue alternating as you move forwards
- Although you can turn around when you've reached the end of your space, practise reversing the movement and crawling backwards

While looking forwards is important for locomotion, it's not necessary if this movement is being performed in a controlled space, e.g. exercise studio, garden etc. If the exercise is being performed as part of a complex movement sequence, then adopting a forward gaze is encouraged.

Progressions: see exercises 8.16, 8.17 and 8.18

Exercise **8.16** Monster walk

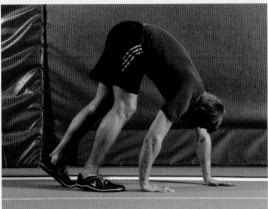

(a) 4-point   (b) 2-point

The higher hip position in this exercise places more demands on the shoulder joint and girdle, and is also dependent on flexibility in the posterior chain (particularly the hamstrings). The set up is the same as in the basic prone crawl, however, the legs are now as straight as possible.

Basic movement

- Begin the crawl as previously described, leading with the arms, before stepping legs forwards
- Note that you will not be able to look forwards when performing this exercise, so ensure you have a clear space ahead of you

Exercise 8.17 Lizard crawl

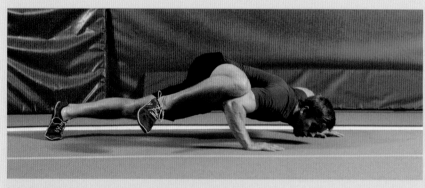

(a) 4-point

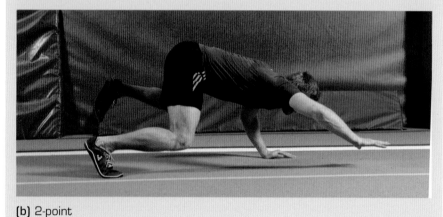

(b) 2-point

While this is a challenging crawling progression, from a movement perspective it sits between the commando crawl and the prone crawl. The challenge arises from the eccentric muscular effort required to perform the exercise, as well as the additional frontal/transverse plane core stabilisation demands.

Basic movement
- Assume a front support position and drop about halfway down into a push-up and hold

- Maintaining this bent elbow position, slide the left arm forwards immediately followed by the right foot – as with the commando crawl, the right knee will move up the side of the body to hip level
- Repeat on the other side, and continue to alternate. This exercise may be regressed by resting on the forearms (as in the commando crawl) with the hips and legs off the ground

Exercise 8.18 Side shuffle

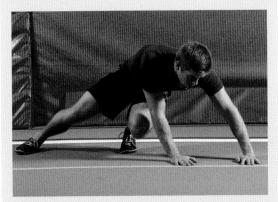

(a) Reach

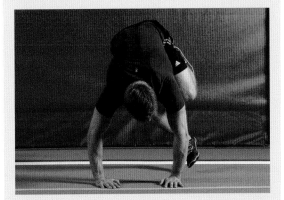

(b) Jump

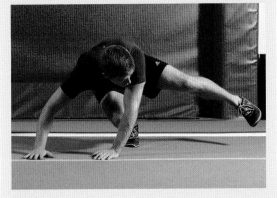

(c) Land

Basic movement

- Begin in the prone crawl position
- Lean your bodyweight into your shoulders/ arms and jump the legs to the left, just past your left hand
- Immediately lift the hands, place them to the left of your legs, and jump the legs across again
- Repeat continuously before swapping directions

The exercise can be modified by stepping the feet across, instead of jumping. This should be a quick stepping/shuffling movement, e.g. if moving to the right, the left foot will step first just before the right foot. Visually, this creates more fluidity of movement.

Exercise 8.19 Crab walk

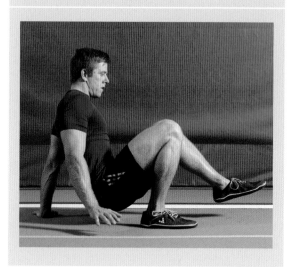

The crab walk is a simple locomotor pattern in the supine position using the hands and feet that can be sequenced well alongside other locomotor patterns.

Basic movement

- Begin in a seated position with knees bent to 90° and feet flat on the floor
- The hands are flat on the floor just behind (and to the outside of) the hips
- The shoulder should be externally rotated which will afford better stability and the fingers should be facing backwards as far as comfortable to help drive the centre of mass forwards during movement
- From this start position, engage the shoulder stabilisers and lift the hips slightly off the floor
- Begin to walk forwards using an opposite arm/leg action

Fluidity of movement

Many advocates of crawling patterns will often promote simultaneous movement of the opposite arm and leg during contralateral patterns. Such an approach will often require excessive core stabilisation, ultimately manifesting in movement stiffness and a loss of fluidity and natural aesthetic.

When observing young children crawling (as well as the locomotion of animals), the limbs move in a clear sequence, usually involving stepping out with the leading limb before moving the opposite trailing limb. Using the basic crawl as an example, the movement is initiated by reaching the right arm forwards and placing it on the floor immediately followed by the left leg moving forward. This sequential, alternating motion of opposing limbs helps to produce an efficient forward movement of the body's centre of mass, while allowing optimal stability and fluidity of movement. It's also important when learning and teaching primitive crawling patterns to think of sequential movement of the opposing limbs – in prone patterns, the arms will lead, and in supine patterns such as the crab walk, the legs will lead.

Exercise 8.20 Shrimping

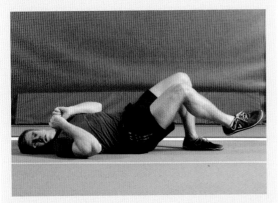

(a) Start position

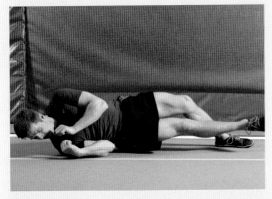

(b) Push off

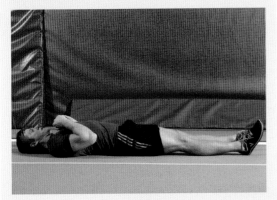

(c) End position

While the art of shrimping is best left to the disciplines of mixed martial arts, the basic movement pattern is an excellent whole body-conditioning exercise performed in the supine position.

Basic movement

- Lie on your back and bend the knees so the feet are close to the buttocks
- Keep the arms and hands in a guard position
- Turn the hips to the right, and immediately press the left foot into the floor as you extend the spine and bridge the left hip slightly
- Continue to push the left foot into the floor, sliding the body backwards until both legs are straight, and the body is in a side-lying flexed position
- Quickly walk the feet back as you roll on to your back and repeat on the other side, alternating continuously
- As a variation, shrimping may be performed on one side before switching to the opposite side; the exercise can also be performed in the seated position

SWEEPS

Sweeps have traditionally been essential movements in combat, and not usually considered to be locomotor patterns. However, as the sweep moves the body horizontally from one point to another it's been included here. Outside of combat, it's an excellent conditioning movement that trains balance, spatial awareness and coordination; it also serves as a useful movement when you need to transition smoothly between the ground and standing. Here we shall focus on the back sweep.

Exercise 8.21 Back sweep

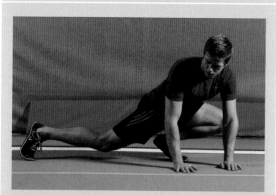

(a) Start position

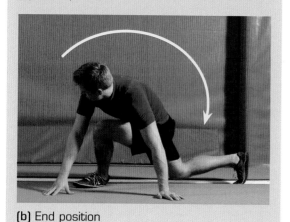

(b) End position

Basic movement

During the back sweep, aim to keep the hips as low to the ground as possible – not only will this enhance stability and balance, it will help to protect the knee joint. To generate more power in the sweep, try to get your bodyweight further over the pivot leg – this may involve placing the hands a little further out, but will help to shift weight off the sweeping leg. Finally, don't forget to drive the same side shoulder to assist the sweep. If you are performing several sweeps as a conditioning drill, keep the hips close to the ground as you perform them; if you are performing the sweep as a transition to an upright position, try to spiral up and out of the movement, so you are ready to flow into the next exercise.

- Assume a deep lunge position with the left leg leading
- Drop deeper into the lunge as you reach down and place the right hand on the floor to the inside of the left foot
- Keeping the right leg straight, pivot on the ball of the left foot and sweep the right leg behind the body until facing the opposite direction
- As you sweep the right leg, switch the right hand for the left as the body rotates – the right hand will naturally come off the floor as you complete the movement
- Continue the back sweep by shifting your weight on to the right leg and sweeping behind with the left

TUMBLING

Tumbling skills are commonly found in the repertoire of gymnasts, acrobats, martial artists, dancers and free runners, however there are two accessible movements that are straightforward to master for those wishing to challenge their bodyweight training: rolling and cartwheels. Both of these movements require the body to be inverted, which helps to develop balance and spatial awareness. These skills can also be programmed into longer movement sequences.

ROLLING BASICS

Rolling is a basic and fundamental gymnastic movement, which has many variations. As well as being a challenging locomotor skill, proper rolling can also help to dissipate the force of a fall. Within a bodyweight training sequence, rolls can be effectively used to link movements together to maintain momentum and flow, or to create power going into a movement.

Exercise 8.22 Forward roll

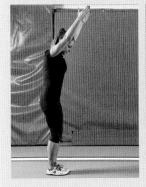 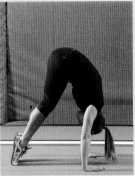 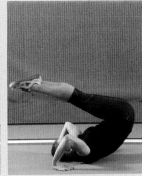 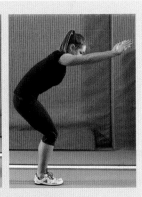

(a) Start   (b) Inverted   (c) Tuck and roll   (d) Finish

- From standing, crouch down and place your hands in front of you on the floor, shoulder width apart (fingers facing forwards)
- Tuck the chin into the chest and place the back of the head/neck on the floor
- Keep bodyweight supported by the arms as you push off the floor with the legs, rotating over the head on to your back

- Keeping the legs tucked, press the feet into the floor, and rapidly reach the arms forwards and upwards to stand
- The return to standing should be performed without placing the hands on the floor – this can be drilled in the deep squat position, rolling back, and explosively reaching forwards with the arms to return to the squat position

Exercise 8.23 Dive forward roll

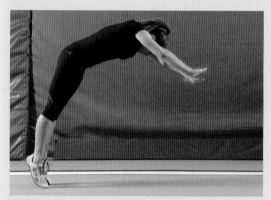

(a) Dive

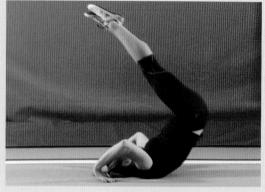

(b) Tuck

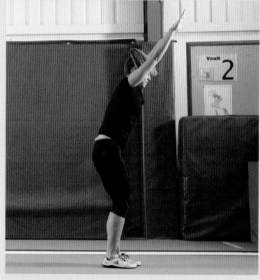

(c) Finish

- Begin this progression from standing, before attempting it with a run up
- From standing, place arms overhead and punch forward off both feet
- The chin should be tucked into the chest as the hands contact the floor some way in front of you
- As you enter this momentary flight phase, maintain a hollow body shape with straight legs
- Complete the forward roll and return to standing

Exercise 8.24 Forward shoulder roll

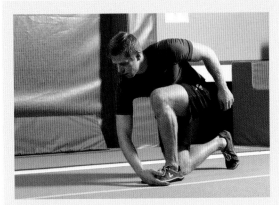

(a) Start

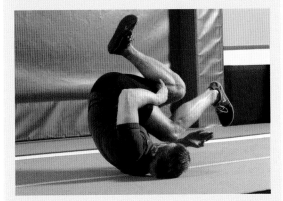

(b) Inverted

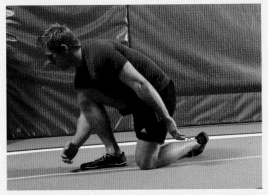

(c) Finish

The shoulder roll is a roll variation that is traditionally used as a safety roll to help break falls and protect the head. However, the mechanics of the roll allow for little loss of momentum, which can be useful during complex movement sequences.

Basic movement

- Begin in a kneeling lunge position, left leg forwards
- Place the right hand on the floor next to the left foot, fingers pointing inwards
- Push off the back foot and roll across the left arm and shoulder
- Keep the legs in a relaxed tuck as you roll over back into the start position. Repeat on the other side
- The roll can be progressed into the standing position, making it more accessible as part of other movements, e.g. landing from a jump and rolling out into a run

Exercise 8.25 Backward shoulder roll

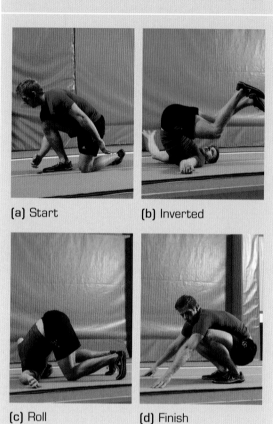

(a) Start

(b) Inverted

(c) Roll

(d) Finish

This is similar to a backward roll except the roll is performed over one shoulder. The backward shoulder roll is a faster movement than the backward roll, and as such may be useful as a linking movement within a complex bodyweight sequence.

Cartwheel

The cartwheel is another fundamental gymnastic skill that involves a sideways rotation of the body. During the move the body moves sideways in a straight line, placing the same side hand on the ground followed by the other hand as the legs move over the head, and return to standing. As well as being a challenging whole body exercise, the cartwheel is also a useful linking movement in bodyweight sequences, e.g. forward roll into cartwheel into running.

Exercise 8.26 Side to side cartwheel

In this cartwheel, you'll start and end in the same position.

- Begin in a standing position with arms overhead and feet shoulder width apart
- Choose the direction in which you are going
- Turn the foot of the lead leg out so that the toes are facing the direction you are going
- Reach down and across the body to plant the lead hand on the ground in front of the lead foot – as you do this, the rear leg should be coming up
- The rear hand will land on the floor just after the lead hand, shoulder width apart
- As the second hand comes down, powerfully kick up the lead leg to bring both legs into a straddle position in the air
- The legs should continue moving forwards in this position, swinging down past the second hand, landing on the rear leg first, then the lead leg
- Ensure that you land with soft knees. The hands will also leave the floor, starting with the lead hand, followed by the rear hand, as you return to the start position
- As a general rule for hand/foot placement, think – hand, hand, foot, foot

Exercise 8.26 Side to side cartwheel

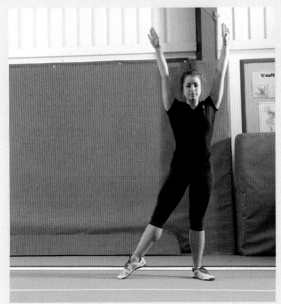

(a) Start position

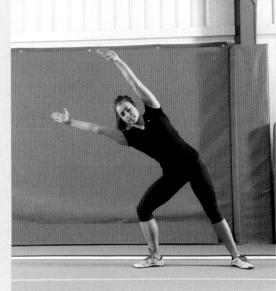

(b) Lunge and reach

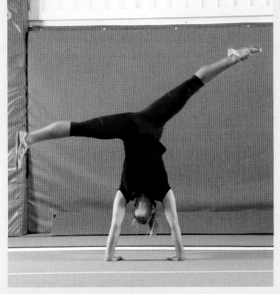

(c) Inverted position

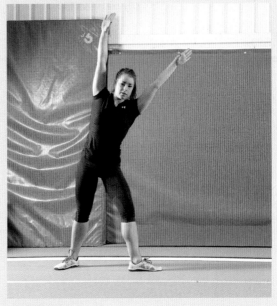

(d) Step out

Exercise 8.27 Front to back cartwheel

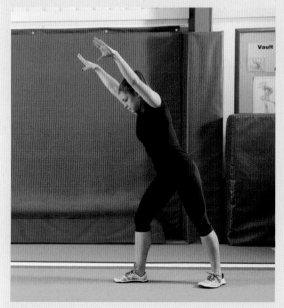

(a) Start position

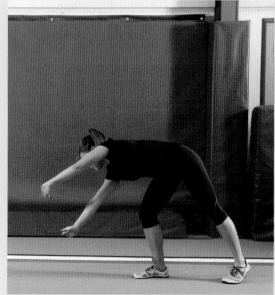

(b) Lunge and reach

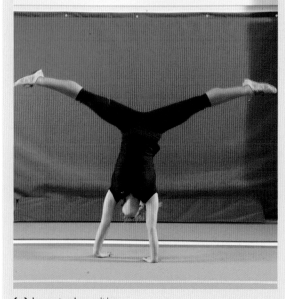

(c) Inverted position

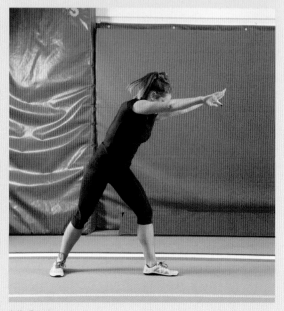

(d) Step out

Exercise 8.27 Front to back cartwheel

In this cartwheel, you start facing forwards, and end up facing backwards – this is the classic gymnastics variation and involves more rotation.

Basic movement

- Begin in a standing position with arms overhead, lunge forwards
- Push off the lead leg and place the first hand on the ground in front of this leg, while simultaneously raising the rear leg
- To better prepare for the rotation, place the second hand next to the first but with the fingers pointing backward, and explosively kick up the rear leg
- Continue through the straddle position, and use your arms to push off the ground
- Straighten your body back into a lunge as your legs swing down one at a time
- You should now have your arms above your head and be facing the opposite direction you originally started in.

Handstand walking

Handstand walking is technically a locomotor pattern and is often mastered before a static handstand is achieved. When performing a handstand walk, it's important to maintain a straight, rigid body, with toes pointed – this helps to create midline stability that will allow you to quickly adjust your posture when necessary. Many beginners will also overarch their spines to initiate a forward lean as a means of propulsion. While this is not wrong, it does create a bad postural habit. In addition, this over-reliance on gravitational torque (i.e. forward lean) will increase the amount of muscular effort required to maintain a controlled walk. Instead, forward propulsion should be driven by hip extension, combined with lifting one hand at a time. It may help to think of the movement as 'walking with the shoulder girdle', rather than walking with the arms.

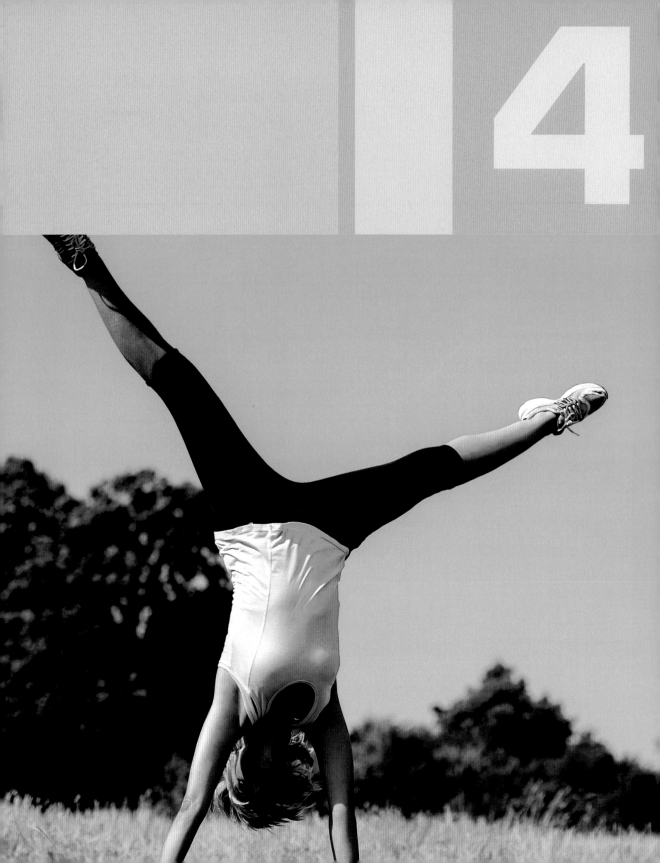

PART **FOUR**

MOVEMENT SEQUENCES AND FLOWS

Now that you've developed a good foundation of strength, balance and coordination using stability, manipulative and locomotor patterns, these individual skills can be combined into progressive and imaginative workouts that are physically challenging, scalable and fun. There are two types of movement sequence to consider when it comes to fitness training: those that are primarily transitional, and those that are more locomotive in nature.

The chapter on transitional sequences focuses on moving efficiently between different body positions with little horizontal (and vertical) displacement. This makes these exercises perfectly suited to environments where space is limited (e.g. at home). Repetition and slow tempo of movement can be used as a progressive tool,

however, some combos may be better suited to faster tempos – generally the larger the transition between successive exercises (i.e. floor to standing position), the faster (and more plyometric) the movement will become. In any case, the aim is to move as fluidly as possible from one to the next.

Sequences that are more locomotive in nature are explored in chapter 8, locomotor sequences, and will usually involve using two or more exercises in a sequence (or flow) that enables the body to move across a greater distance (usually horizontally). These sequences therefore allow for continuous repetition (space permitting), and will often bring about greater cardiovascular effort and demand more muscular endurance. These types of movement are best suited for larger spaces, such as gardens, parks or exercise studios. In a fully integrated bodyweight session, transitional and locomotor sequences can be combined to produce an imaginative and playful workout.

It's worth noting that there are a number of movement and fitness training disciplines in existence that inspire the natural, playful and developmental aspect of bodyweight movement sequences, including Parkour, capoeira, Animal Flow, Body Flow, and Ginastica Natural – their underlying philosophies may help the fitness enthusiast to explore new ideas and directions in their bodyweight training routines.

Whether the movement sequence is transitional or locomotive in nature, it's important to execute it with efficiency and economy of effort. This will result in movement that is skilful and balanced, as well as aesthetically appealing. Building a strong foundation in the stability, manipulative, and locomotor patterns will ensure that these movements are performed with skill; improvements in mobility, balance, strength, endurance and power will naturally follow on from this.

The transitional and locomotor sequences that follow will focus on short combinations of exercises, and are by no means exhaustive. However, they will provide a number of ideas on how to move into and out of different bodyweight exercises efficiently. Central to fluid movement is learning how to make the correct body shape, as well as how to generate and take advantage of momentum. As you learn to use momentum to your advantage through regular practice of these basic sequences, you will no doubt discover new and innovative ways to sequence movement. Most importantly, as your skill in the building block exercises increases, so too will your execution of movement sequences, as you learn how to manipulate your body efficiently through space.

TRANSITIONAL SEQUENCES

Transitional sequences focus on seamlessly moving from one body shape and/or position to another, and do not involve large amounts of horizontal movement. In theory, almost any combination of two or more exercises can be sequenced; however, in reality, a smooth transition between each may not be immediately apparent, and may warrant further exploration.

Each of the sequences described below are made up of two or more exercises – mostly stability and manipulative skills. It's important to understand that these sequences will demand higher levels of dynamic stabilisation, muscular endurance and power, especially when performed under repetition.

1. Hollow to super hero
2. Under switch
3. Over switch
4. Front support to crow
5. Push-up to stand
6. Crab to stand
7. Burpee
8. Kick through
9. Candlestick
10. Muscle-up.

These sequences have been chosen to showcase the simplicity, diversity and scalability of bodyweight training, and are by no means exhaustive. When performing these exercises, it's important not to think of them in terms of muscles worked, but instead the movement skill being taught. While the intention of these exercises is to develop fitness, explore ways in which these movement skills can be transferred to other exercises, as well as daily activities. In any case, you are strongly encouraged to further explore the building block movements in earlier sections, as well as the disciplines of gymnastics, dance, Parkour and mixed martial arts for further ideas.

Tip

It will be assumed that the component exercises contained within each sequence have been mastered; therefore, their individual instruction will not be covered in great detail here. However, each sequence will explore variations and experimental movements that the bodyweight enthusiast can use to both challenge and stylise their training.

Exercise 9.1 Hollow to super hero

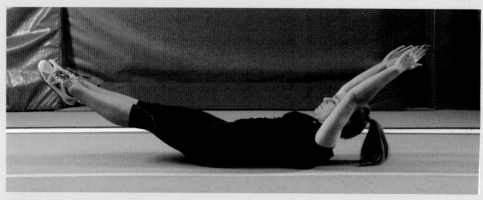

(a) Start

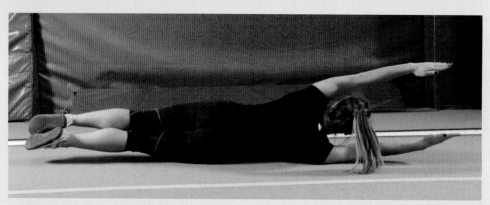

(b) Roll

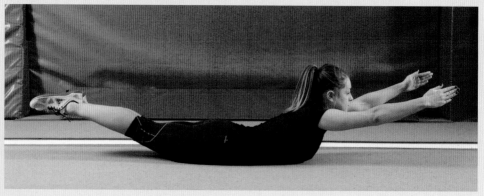

(c) End

This short movement is a perfect example of how two simple static exercises can be combined to create a sequence that requires a high level of stabilisation, strength and coordination. While the hollow hold and super hero positions have been previously explored, the challenge in this sequence is the efficient transition between the two. For this reason, it's an excellent conditioning drill for training body tension and midline stability, that is transferable to almost every other bodyweight exercise.

Basic movement

- Assume a hollow body hold with the arms overhead and toes pointed away
- Keep the glutes and quads engaged, and get a sense of the amount of body tension required to maintain this shape
- Without losing tension, roll the entire body into the super hero position and hold
- Return to the start position and repeat on the other side

Further explorations

- If space permits, complete several continuous rolls in one direction, before rolling back in the opposite direction.
- The initial roll to the super hero position can be explored in a number of ways. Try creating a drive from the hips – think about lifting the opposite side hip to drive the movement. Alternatively, explore lifting (and turning) the head and chest back (cervical/thoracic extension) to drive the roll. Finally, explore the strategy used by babies and initiate the roll by turning the eyes in the direction of the movement.

- The roll from super hero back to a hollow position can be explored in a similar way. In this position, the muscular effort required (and limited mobility in the lumbar spine) to rotate the body back to the hollow position can be challenging. Instead, try to exploit the available mobility in the cervical/thoracic spine. For example if trying to rotate to the left, reach up the floor with the left arm and simultaneously pull the left arm down, pushing the left shoulder behind and to the left: this counter-movement with the arms will produce a spinal rotation that will help drive the entire body back to the hollow position.
- Experiment with different body shapes once you have mastered the basic movement. Although torso stability should be maintained throughout the roll, try different arm and leg positions. For example, in the hollow position, keep the left arm overhead but hold the right hand by your chest. Now scissor the right leg over the left leg to drive a roll to the left – this will create a faster roll to the super hero position. As you land in the super hero position, your right hand should be under the chest, palm down. From here, a quick pull down of the left hand will put both hands in a position where you can perform a push-up, or an explosive push-up to standing; alternatively, you can simply reverse the movement and roll back to the start position.

Exercise 9.2 Under switch

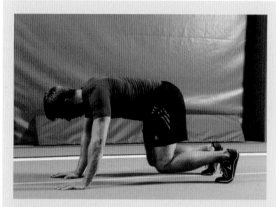

(a) Start position

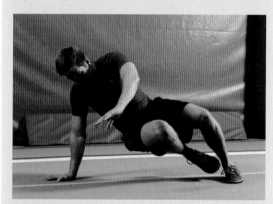

(b) Hip drive

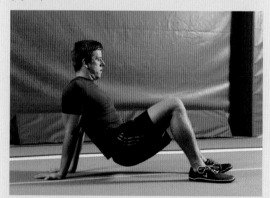

(c) End position

This simple yet elegant switching movement efficiently moves the body from a crawl to a crab position, by rotating the hips underneath the torso. Although it requires less muscular effort compared to other bodyweight exercises, it's a useful exercise for improving shoulder and hip mobility, and for quickly transitioning between prone and supine positions.

Basic movement

- From a prone crawl position, drive the right hip underneath the torso towards the left, pivoting on the left foot
- As the right knee crosses the body, raise the left arm by driving the left shoulder back
- Simultaneously place the left hand on the floor underneath the left shoulder and place the right foot next to the left foot
- If you imagine starting from a 12 o'clock position on a clock face, you should now be facing 5 o'clock
- Reverse the movement by pulling the right leg through, reaching back with the left arm, and pivoting on the left foot
- Repeat to the other side

Further explorations

- This exercise can be used as part of a warm-up to help drill hip rotation and shoulder flexibility
- This movement now links the prone crawl to the crab walk, so explore switching between the two as smoothly as possible

Exercise 9.3 Over switch

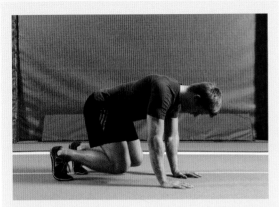

(a) Start position

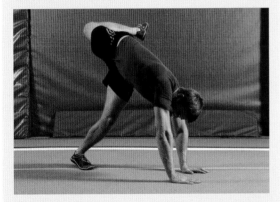

(b) Hip drive

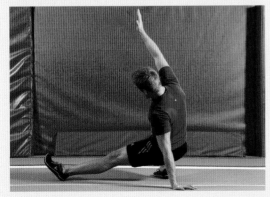

(c) End position

The over-switch movement provides a similar transition from prone to supine as the under switch, except the hips rotate behind and over the torso. This movement is also known as the scorpion, or scorpion kick.

Basic movement
- From a prone crawl position straighten the left leg and push the hips upwards
- Simultaneously, reach the right foot behind the body towards the opposite shoulder – this will open up the right hip and begin the rotation
- As you continue to reach the right leg behind the body, start to lift the right arm off the floor and slowly drive the right shoulder in the same direction as the right leg
- As the chest begins to open up, turn the head to face the opposite direction, as you plant the right foot and right hand on the floor
- Pull the left leg in to complete the crab position

Further explorations
- The over switch also links the prone crawl to the crab walk, so explore switching between the two as smoothly as possible. Other ideas to try include the over switch straight into a kick to stand (see back support to stand); or perform a drop to push-up, into an over switch, followed by a candlestick roll to standing.
- To challenge mobility and coordination further, begin in a crab position and perform an under switch into a prone crawl position. Without planting the foot on the floor immediately perform an over switch using the same leg. In this exploration, you are effectively rotating the torso 360° – if performed correctly, you should end up facing the same direction, but slightly further across the floor.

Exercise 9.4 Front support to crow

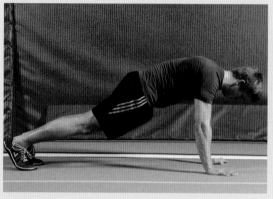

(a) Start)

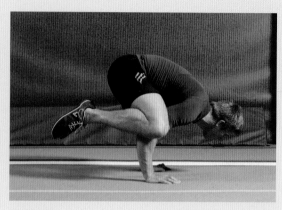

(b) Finish

This exercise involves moving quickly from one isometric hold to another, and challenges endurance, strength, coordination and balance.

Basic movement

- Assume a front support position and engage the glutes and quads
- Keeping the arms straight, lean back into the legs bending the knees slightly to load
- Immediately unload from this position by quickly lifting the hips up and pulling the knees to the outside of the elbows
- Rapidly engage the core and shoulders to decelerate as you balance the knees on the outside of the elbows
- Hold the crow position for a few seconds, before jumping back to front support

Further explorations

- Before performing the exercise it may be useful to assume the crow position first – this will 'groove' the correct muscle-activation patterns and aid muscle memory
- Try loading the hips and legs more by bending further back into a crouch position. This will consequently require more deceleration and stabilisation when jumping into the crow hold, adding intensity to the exercise. For a different challenge, try reducing the loading phase to as little as possible, i.e. jumping from a static front support into the crow
- Add speed to the movement, smoothly jumping from one position to the other with no holds
- Think about linking other exercises, for example, adding a push-up or prone crawl before the front support; or performing the inch-worm exercise in between the holds

Exercise 9.5 Push-up to stand

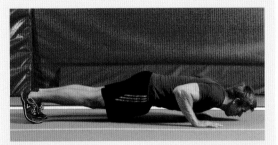

(a) Start

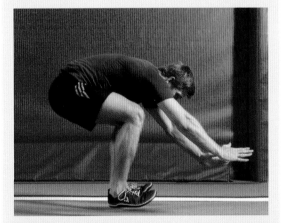

(b) Explode and tuck

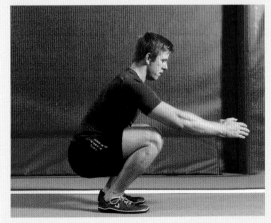

(c) Finish

As well as being an excellent conditioning exercise for power, the push-up to stand is also useful when you need to quickly move from lying to upright.

Basic movement

Begin in a front support position and drop down into a push-up. As soon as you hit the lowest position, explosively push up while simultaneously pulling the knees to the chest. As your feet approach your hands, kick the legs out and plant the feet, pulling the arms off the floor and landing in a balanced squat position before standing straight.

Further explorations

- Variations may include push-up to single leg balance, and push-up to lunge.
- It's important to understand that this exercise is about creating rotation quickly and efficiently, and this is dependent on forming the correct body shape – a tuck position. To achieve this, begin the push-up by lifting the chest – this will create an extension force in the posterior muscles, and begin to load up the hip and trunk flexors. As soon as you sense the trunk muscles beginning to stretch, explosively flex the trunk (pull the belly upwards) and drive the hips underneath you. To maximise the rotation, try to lift the hands off the floor before the feet land – this will limit the amount of torque and consequent muscular effort.
- The push-up to stand can be easily linked to any movement that uses the front support. For example, the front support roll to push-up to stand; or simply adding the jump to stand after a set of push-ups, or crawling patterns. Any standing exercise can be linked to the end of this exercise, for example, push-up to single leg balance into a pistol squat.

Exercise **9.6** Crab to stand

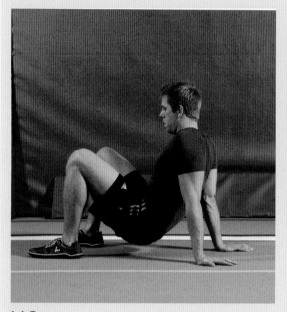

(a) Start

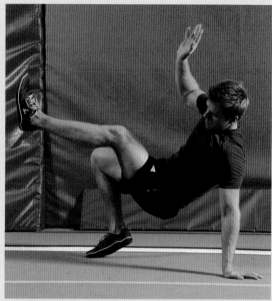

(b) Hip drive

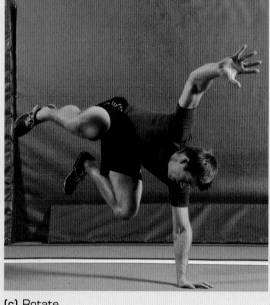

(c) Rotate

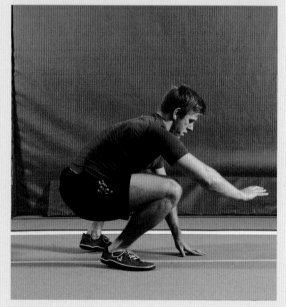

(d) Finish

While the push-up to stand focuses on transitioning from prone to standing, the crab to stand offers a solution from supine. Correct technique requires full single arm bodyweight support, rapid hip extension/rotation, as well as good shoulder joint flexibility – a thorough warm-up of these areas is strongly recommended.

Basic movement

- Assume a crab position with arms straight
- Lift the left leg off the floor slightly and raise the right arm in front of you – these two limbs will be the initial driver for the movement
- When ready, kick the left leg up and press the right foot into the floor to rapidly extend the hip
- As the hip moves upwards, quickly lift the right leg and pull it across the body to the left
- At the same time, keep the core engaged as you drive the right shoulder to the left, rotating your torso around the left shoulder to face backwards
- As your body rotates, the left foot should land first, quickly followed by the right foot – with the body ending up facing the opposite direction in a deep squat
- Repeat on the other side

Further explorations

The coordination of this movement is often the most challenging part, but the sequence can be broken down and drilled to improve awareness and position sense.

- Firstly, hand placement is essential to minimise risk of over-exertion and injury. In the crab position, ensure that the fingers of the support hand are pointing backwards – this requires a good level of external rotation at the shoulder; regular practise of the back support exercise will improve mobility and flexibility in the shoulder.
- The next step is the hip drive, which can be explored in two ways. From the crab position, try dropping the hips to the floor before kicking the leg up – this will tap into the elastic potential of the posterior chain to maximise rapid hip extension. Pushing the right foot into the floor to actively assist hip extension is also key.
- Scissor kick – the action of the left leg kick, immediately followed by the right leg is effectively a scissor kick. This can be practised as a standalone drill in standing or in the crab position.
- Torso rotation – the final step involves torso rotation which is driven by the right hip and right shoulder (in this example). The scissor kick will begin the rotation to the left, so it's important to drive the right shoulder to the left also, swinging the right arm around as if trying to reach the floor behind you. As the torso rotates, try pushing the left hand hard into the ground – as well as creating a stable anchor point, it will also help to create lift.

Once mastered, explore ways to link this to other movements. For example, try a crab walk then jump out to standing; a push-up, followed by a roll to back support, into a crab, then jump to stand; or a deep squat into crab position, into a jump to stand, and repeat on the other side.

Exercise 9.7 Burpee

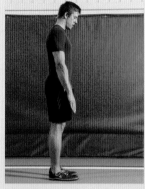

(a) Start

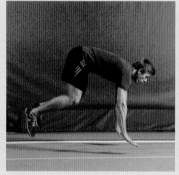

(b) Jump to push-up

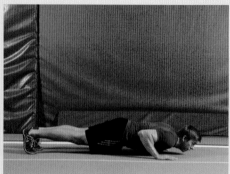

(c) Bottom of push-up

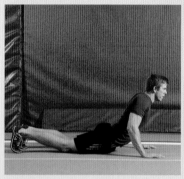

(d) Extend

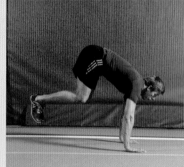

(e) Explode and tuck

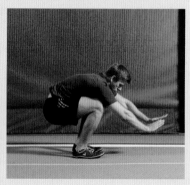

(f) Stand

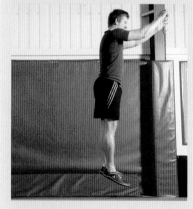

(g) Jump

The burpee has long been a favourite drill in strength training circles. In more recent times, the growth of training systems such as CrossFit and military fitness has cemented its position as a popular whole body metabolic conditioning exercise that develops strength, endurance, power, coordination and cardiovascular fitness.

Basic movement

From a standing position, squat down and place your hands just in front of your feet. Immediately kick the legs back to front support and perform a push-up. Explode out of the push-up into a squat and immediately jump up, landing back in the start position.

Further explorations

The key to a successful burpee is speed, which will allow the body to maximise its elastic potential and minimise unnecessary muscular effort. Once you can perform the burpee as a stepped sequence (i.e. squat to push-up to squat to jump) you can explore adding speed to link the individual movements together as follows:

- Practise 'jumping' into the push-up. Begin by looking at where your feet are − this is where you will place your hands. From standing, start to drop into the squat position, and as your hands get nearer to the floor, kick out the legs and catch yourself in front support (hands where feet were). As soon as you catch yourself, allow the body to drop into a push-up, using elasticity to rebound into the front support.

Drill this sequence many times to get a feel for correct hand placement and awareness of decelerating the body. Because the jump into the push-up involves a short flight phase (all limbs off the ground) it can initially be a little daunting to try this. A softer surface, such as several mats, or a crash mat, may help increase confidence in catching yourself and decelerating towards the floor. It's also worth noting that some burpee purists may frown upon jumping into the push-up, as it partly eliminates the squat movement; however, as a skill-based conditioning drill, it's highly effective.

- The next step is to maximise elasticity during the push-up to squat. A successful return to the standing position is dependent on rapid displacement of the body's centre of mass (upward hip drive), as well as efficient rotation (knee tuck and arm swing). Please refer to the 'push-up to stand' exercise for a detailed explanation of this movement.
- The final step of the burpee progression is the squat to jump. As you jump into the squat from the push-up, try punching the floor with the feet as you land to create a rebound into the jump; alternatively, the moment you land the squat, bounce into it a little to maximise elastic recoil for the jump.
- Practise putting the above steps together, focusing on a seamless transition between them. Master the skill at lower repetitions with higher rest periods, before increasing repetitions for fitness.

Exercise 9.8 Kick through

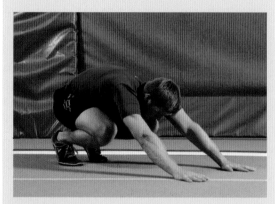

(a) Start

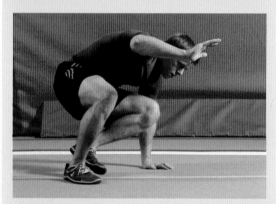

(b) Kick

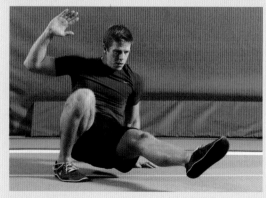

(c) End position

The kick through (and variations of) have been used in mixed martial arts, capoeira and dance for some time, and have more recently gained popularity in fitness training via Mike Fitch's Animal Flow. The movement demands dynamic stability, strength, power and coordination to move the body from a prone to a supine position. The kick through can be drilled on its own, or integrated as part of a continuous movement sequence.

Basic movement

- Begin in a prone crawl position, arms straight and knees bent
- Keeping the hands where they are, sit back into a crouch, engage the abdominals, and immediately jump the feet towards the hands
- As you jump, bear your weight through the left arm, while simultaneously lifting the right hand and replacing it with the right foot
- As the right foot lands, kick the left leg through the space between your left hand and right leg
- The end position will have the body supported on the left hand and right leg, with the left leg held straight out in front and the right hand in the guard position
- Reverse the movement by quickly pulling the left leg back, driving the hips upwards, and jumping back to the crouch/crawl position
- Repeat on the other side

Further explorations

- If the full kick through is initially challenging, the movement can be simplified into the step to kick through, which will help to drill body awareness. In this version, instead of jumping the legs through from a crouch/crawl position, step the right foot forward and place it next to the right hand. Quickly lift the right hand as you kick through the left leg. As your positional awareness and stability improve, progressively add speed, ultimately building up to the jump to kick through.

- The side kick through is a subtle variation of the (forward) kick through, and relies on driving the hip through rotation. From the prone crawl position, drive the left hip underneath the body to the right, pivoting on the right foot as you do. As the left knee comes across the body, lift the right hand and kick the left leg out to the right. You will now be facing to the right. Return to the start position and repeat on the other side. As you improve, add a small jump to the kick through. For added intensity, try jumping and kicking through 180° from right to left (i.e. no return to the crawl position.

- A number of other movements can be added before and after the kick through, both for added intensity and diversity of movement. In all cases, try to maintain fluidity and control of movement. For example, the kick through can be preceded by prone crawling, adding a kick through to each side every few steps; for a high power sequence, try the burpee kick through – from standing, drop into the push-up, explode into a kick through, jump back to a push-up, and jump to standing. Repeat and alternate legs with the kick through. Also, think about exercises that can be added on to the end of a kick through. For example, jumping into a stand (see back support to stand), or a simple rotation out back into a prone crawl position (see crawl to crab switch).

Exercise 9.9 Candlestick

(a) Start

(b) Roll back

(c) Shoulder stand

(d) Roll forward

(e) Finish

The candlestick is another fundamental gymnastics skill that develops mobility, balance, and coordination, which can be transferred to other skills such as rolling. From a conditioning perspective, it's a highly effective core exercise, and provides yet another way of moving between the ground and upright standing. The candlestick sequence combines a squat, backward roll, and shoulder stand, and should be performed continuously with speed.

Basic movement

- Stand tall with feet together, glutes and abdominals engaged
- Push the hips back as you drop into a deep squat. At the bottom of the squat, continue the movement with a controlled fall backwards into a backward roll
- As you roll, extend the arms overhead and drive the hips up and straighten the legs into a shoulder stand position – pause momentarily
- Keeping the abdominals engaged, use the momentum generated to roll back down maintaining a hollow body shape – as soon as the low back makes contact with the ground, simultaneously pull the feet in and explosively reach forwards with the arms to drive back into a squat
- Drive the hips forward and up to return to the start position.

Further explorations

- Efficient execution of this movement is highly dependent on both shoulder flexibility and the ability to maintain a tight hollow shape. Limited range of motion in shoulder extension may result in flattening of the thoraco-lumbar spine, which will inhibit spinal motion and cause a loss of momentum during the roll. If the hollow shape is weak, there is often a tendency to try and 'kick out' of the movement too early, and/or excessively contract the abdominals in an attempt to drive back to the squat position. With this in mind, the hollow hold and hollow rock are prerequisite conditioning drills for the candlestick.
- The single leg candlestick offers an interesting progression that further challenges balance.

The candlestick is performed in the usual way, except that the return to the squat position occurs on a single leg. It's worth noting that a return to a single leg stance will allow you to step out of the movement and continue the flow of movement, for example, adding a cartwheel afterwards, or even dropping into a lunge.

- Explore other exercises that can be added before or after the candlestick to create longer fluid sequences. For a power-based sequence, any type of jump (tuck, straddle, pike, 180°) can be performed before the candlestick; or for a more isometric sequence, begin in the super hero position, roll into a hollow hold, drive up to shoulder stand and roll out to standing.
- An interesting sequence to explore is the burpee to candlestick. While it should be straightforward to perform these two exercises back to back, a simple modification of the burpee will ensure a smooth transition between the two exercises without any loss of momentum. During a burpee, the jump back to a squat position is balanced, i.e. the feet land directly under your centre of mass. When linking the burpee into the candlestick, try to land the feet a little further forward of your centre of mass. At the same time, focus on pulling the arms off the floor and driving them upwards before the feet land. The combination of feet forward and arms driving up will put the body in a position of falling backwards into the candlestick. In a similar way, use the momentum of the candlestick roll up to jump into the push-up portion of the burpee.

Exercise 9.10 Muscle-up

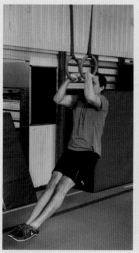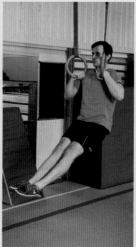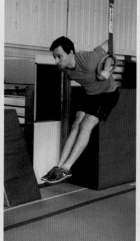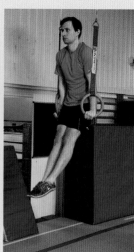

(a) Start   (b) Pull   (c) Transition   (d) Finish

No bodyweight training programme would be complete without the muscle-up – a movement that involves a pull-up immediately followed by a dip. This fundamental gymnastic skill has recently found its way into mainstream fitness as one of the most challenging yet sought after skills, both for its strength and aesthetic appeal. Functionally, this movement also serves as a way of pulling the body up and over an obstacle. Traditionally, the gymnastic muscle-up is performed on the rings, although fixed bar muscle-ups are also popular and highly accessible in gyms and outdoor playgrounds.

Basic movement

- Begin by hanging from the rings in a false grip (palms facing in), and holding a hollow body shape. Don't worry if you cannot fully extend your elbows at this point

- Start to pull yourself upwards, aiming to bring the rings towards the hips – in reality the rings should end up just below the chest, but visualising the hips is a useful cue

- To support this action, try to keep the rings together by squeezing the elbows to the sides, and think about pulling the elbows backwards behind the body. This can be mentally challenging because many will be familiar with pulling the chest forwards during other pulling and rowing exercises. Unfortunately, this strategy will result in the loss of a hollow shape which is key to the muscle-up

- As soon as your hands are just below the chest, it's time for the transition

- Keeping the rings close together and close to the body, the most important thing is getting your shoulders (i.e. your weight) over your hands as quickly as possible. This is done by leaning forward and as quickly as possible rolling the shoulders over the hands (think of an explosive sit-up)

• Simultaneously turn the rings outwards to prepare for the change in hand position as you enter the dip phase

It's worth reiterating the importance of maintaining a tight hollow shape during the transition.

The hollow shape will position the legs slightly in front of the rings at the start, allowing you to remain behind the rings during the pull. During the transition, this tight body shape will rotate more easily around the rings. Following transition, you should find yourself in the bottom of a dip – keep the elbows close to the sides and push up to a straight arm support.

Mastering the false grip

The gymnastics rings muscle-up is dependent on mastering the false grip – which involves placing the wrists above the rings rather than below it. As a result, it requires a higher level of strength in the forearms.

While it's not the most comfortable grip, it is essential for the transition phase of the muscle-up. Initially, the lack of forearm flexibility (and strength) will prevent you from holding a false grip in a fully extended hang – this is why you will see many individuals perform the muscle-up from a partially bent arm position. However, it's worth spending the time and effort in practising this grip, and to allow the forearms to become more flexible, so that eventually you can hold a false grip with full elbow extension (i.e. a dead hang).

• Begin by placing your wrists on the rings, and then flex your hands towards your elbows and towards the inside of the wrists

• With the wrists in this position, wrap your fingers around the top of the rings (thumbs underneath)

• This hand position is difficult to hold at first, so ensure you progressively work on it starting from unloaded (or partially loaded) to full bodyweight loading

Although muscle-ups can be performed with a regular grip, it will require excessive pulling strength as well as a significant kipping action with the legs. There's little to be gained by developing your pulling strength, only to be limited by the strength to hold a false grip. Therefore, practise both at the same time. One way of doing this is to perform false grip body rows on the rings or on a suspension trainer; alternatively, build up endurance and flexibility in your forearms by holding a kettlebell in a false grip.

A small word of warning – the false grip fixes the wrist in one position throughout the exercise, with the pivot point being on the inside of the wrist. As pressure and friction are applied to this area, chafing and minor skin tears may occur which will require time to heal and toughen up. As well as using chalk to minimise friction during muscle-ups, taping around this area may also help, especially when working on volume.

Exercise 9.11 Bar muscle-up

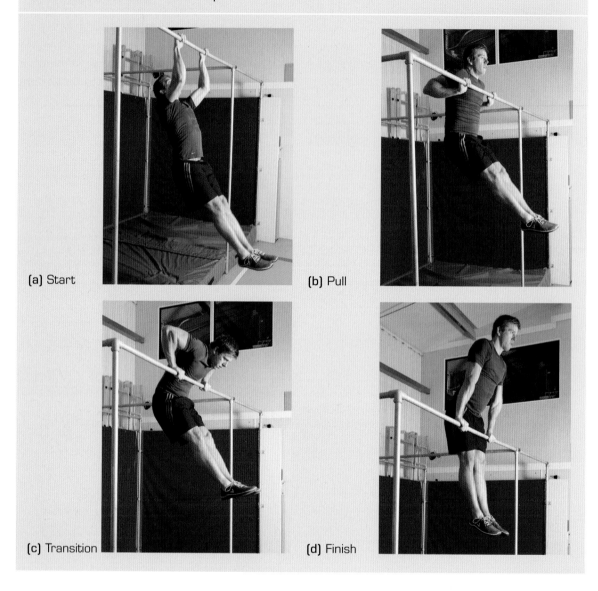

(a) Start

(b) Pull

(c) Transition

(d) Finish

This variation can be performed in several ways, although in the spirit of the rings muscle-up, controlled technique will be described here.

- Start by hanging from a fixed bar with a false grip
- Due to the shape of the bar (compared to the rings) aim to place as much of the wrist on top of the bar as possible

- Using the same technique as the rings, think about pulling the bar towards the hips before rapidly leaning forwards over the hands and bringing the elbows up and over the bar

Very early on in learning the muscle-up you will become aware how challenging this skill is, and will seek out ways to make it easier. One popular method (for the bar muscle-up) is to make the movement faster using a kick or a swing which will allow you to work up to a slow, controlled muscle-up.

- The kick – as you pull up, forcefully kick the legs in front of you (straight legs act as a longer lever, allowing you to generate more lifting power, although bent knees can also be used). Be sure to coordinate the kick with the pull and think about bringing the bar towards the hips. At the transition, quickly lean forwards, getting the shoulders over the hands and the elbows up and over the bar. One last thing to think about is what to do with the legs after the kick up. Keeping the hip slightly flexed (i.e. legs in front of the bar) will assist the rotation; however, keeping them too far in front of the bar will pull you into backward rotation and stop you from getting over the bar.
- The swing – the use of a swing in getting over the bar is also known as a kip in gymnastics, and while it's useful to learn different ways in getting over the bar, many muscle-up purists will regard this as a drastic technique for muscle-ups. Begin by swinging forwards under the bar with arms straight. Then wait until you are at the end of the back-swing before explosively pulling yourself up and over the bar. Note that if you pull too early, you'll be under the bar, and if you pull too late, you'll already be on the down-swing – neither of which will get you over the bar.
- It's important to note that fast muscle-ups using a kick or swing remove the need for a false grip. As you pull yourself up, ensure you get your wrists over the bar, otherwise despite getting the required height, you won't be able to rotate around the bar, and at worst, you may injure your wrists. Chalk on the hands will help to shift the wrists, however with time you'll be able to quickly 'pop' the wrists over the bar.

The rings or bar muscle-up can also be regressed by using a box or step to stand on (or rest the feet on) under the rings or bar. This can be used to either reduce the range of motion in pulling and/or the amount of bodyweight being pulled – allowing you to drill the all-important transition phase. When using a box/step, place it in front of you so that you can rest your heels on it.

Tip

It's a common misconception that the muscle-up requires drilling chin-ups and dips. While a basic level of competency in these exercises is essential, it's not necessary to drill these at high volumes. The key to muscle-up success is good range of extension at the wrist and shoulder joint, and the ability to drive the hips towards the rings. This is followed by optimal rotation around the rings, which is dependent on the maintenance of a tight hollow body position. With this in mind, exercises such as the hollow body hold (and rock), front and back supports are essential conditioning drills, alongside good chin-up and dip technique.

LOCOMOTOR SEQUENCES

Locomotor sequences focus on combinations of locomotor patterns designed to move your body from one point to another. These sequences will predominantly involve large amounts of horizontal displacement, as well as some vertical displacement (e.g. jumping).

Although many of the individual locomotor patterns described in this text will challenge the bodyweight enthusiast, sequencing two or more together will significantly increase requirements for strength, endurance, balance, coordination, agility and spatial awareness. Due to the nature of locomotor patterns, these sequences can offer a different approach to fitness training, rather than simply performing a pre-determined number of sets and repetitions. For example, an exercise studio can be set up with a number of obstacles and the aim is to use a variety of locomotor patterns to move from one end to the other. Parkour and free running are great examples of how different locomotor patterns are used to traverse a particular landscape.

Each of the sequences in this section are made up of two or more locomotor patterns performed back to back as efficiently as possible. This is by no means an exhaustive list, but merely a platform for discovery. When exploring these sequences for yourself, consider linking other bodyweight exercises to add variety and scope. This will also serve to break up the sequence and allow for active rest. As previously mentioned, specific disciplines such as Parkour, Ginastica Natural and capoeira involve artful, intricate and fluid movement sequences that will inspire any bodyweight enthusiast.

For ease of understanding, and to build confidence during learning, the different locomotor sequences will be explored by looking at their starting pattern, as follows:

1. Walking and running sequences
2. Jumping and vaulting sequences
3. Quadrupedal sequences
4. Tumbling sequences.

Tip

It will be assumed that the locomotor patterns contained within each sequence have been mastered; therefore, their individual instruction will not be covered in great detail here. However, each sequence will explore variations and experimental movements that the bodyweight enthusiast can use to both challenge and stylise their training.

WALKING AND RUNNING

Walking and running provide a familiar starting point from which to link efficiently into almost any other locomotor pattern. Walking in particular also has the benefit of providing an active rest when alternated with more challenging patterns, e.g. walk, crawl, walk, crawl etc.

Exercise 10.1 Walk to crawl

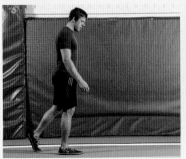

(a) Walk

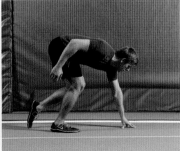

(b) Reach down

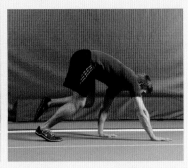

(c) Crawl

Although the walk to crawl is a simple transition, the challenge lies in making the switch as efficiently as possible without breaking the flow of movement.

Basic movement

- From walking, bend the hips and reach down to the floor in front of you with one hand
- Follow this with the other hand, as you bend further into the prone crawl position, and continue alternating with the legs
- To return to walking, step up and out of the movement as one leg comes forward
- Maintain the rhythm as much as possible during transitions

Further explorations

- The key to a good transition is to maintain forward momentum as you move from walking into the crawl and back again. For example, as the left foot strikes during walking, bend the hips and reach the right hand to the floor. Continue to bear weight into the hand and follow up quickly with the left hand. The right foot will naturally follow as you continue the crawl pattern. The return to walking begins as you step forward with one of the feet – simply push through the leg as you come upright, continuing to swing the opposite leg through as you walk.
- The use of a metronome (or music) may help to establish a rhythm. Set the rhythm to 60 bpm and begin walking – one foot strike per beat. Practise the same with the crawling pattern. Now try to move from walking to crawling while still hitting the beat – as the foot strikes on the beat, the opposite hand should immediately hit the floor on the next half beat. The legs will then continue on the beat as you crawl.

Exercise 10.2 Walk to cartwheel

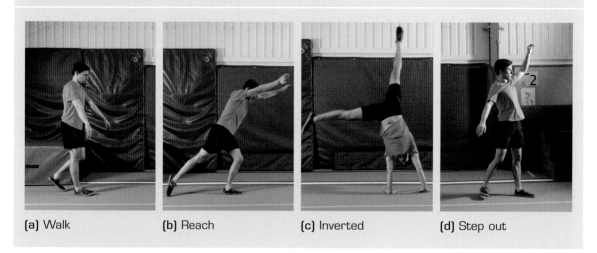

(a) Walk   (b) Reach   (c) Inverted   (d) Step out

The walk to cartwheel is a natural progression from performing a cartwheel from standing.

Basic movement

- Walk a few steps, then as the lead leg starts to swing through, raise the arms overhead
- As the foot strikes the ground, bend the knee, taking your bodyweight over as you reach for the ground with the hands
- Perform the cartwheel and step out
- Immediately pivot on the back leg and rotate the body to face forwards, stepping back into the walk with the opposite leg

Further explorations

- Instead of rotating to face forward out of the cartwheel, you can perform a front to back cartwheel and face backwards. The forward momentum you have generated can then be used to perform a backward roll, or even a candlestick.
- The run into cartwheel variation is a faster variation that will require use of a transitional movement to prepare for the cartwheel – known as a hurdle, or hurdle step. This move not only helps to maintain the flow of the sequence, but is also used to generate speed and power into the cartwheel. When setting up for a cartwheel, the hurdle is a skip on the right leg just before you lunge forwards with the left leg. It's important to note that the run into cartwheel will generate a larger amount of speed coming out of the movement, and it's important to think about where to direct that momentum, rather than coming to a complete stop. If you are looking to continue with running, come out of the cartwheel and immediately perform a jump-half turn with a small skip to face forwards, and fall back into the running pattern. Alternatively, you could do a jump-half turn into a dive forward roll – this would then give you the option of stepping out into a run, or staying on the ground and performing a crawl pattern.

Exercise 10.3 Run to dive forward roll

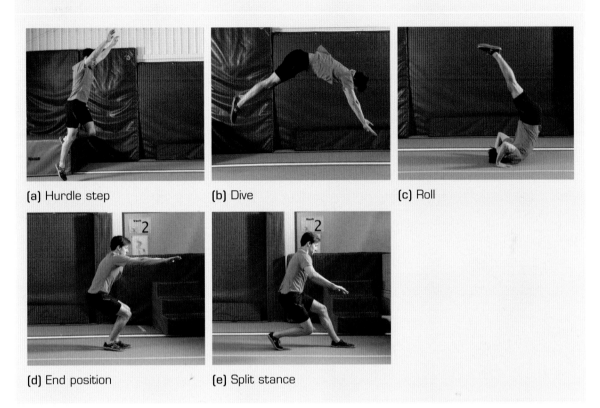

(a) Hurdle step   (b) Dive   (c) Roll

(d) End position   (e) Split stance

The run to dive forward roll is a visually stunning movement due to the flight phase (hands and feet leave the ground). As well as being a highly skilled movement and training drill, functionally, it can be used as an alternative to jumping over low objects.

Basic movement

As with the run to cartwheel, a hurdle will be required to ensure a smooth transition. In this case, the hurdle will be from one foot to two feet.

- As you run up, skip on the right leg while stretching the left leg forwards
- Immediately swing the right leg through to join the left, and plant both into the ground for a double leg take off into the dive forward roll
- Execute the dive roll, and step out one leg at a time to continue running

Further explorations

- During the hurdle, try to punch the ground hard with both feet as you take off. Keep the knees slightly bent as you punch, and extend to straight legs during the dive. The punch will help to translate forward momentum into vertical momentum, which is required if you want to get more height in the dive.

- When running outside on grass or softer trails, look for opportunities where you can add a dive roll, e.g. over a small object such as a log. To maintain the flow of movement, use a single leg take off to dive into the roll, and come out into a split stance to continue the run.
- Because of the speed generated through this movement, the transition back into a run

will offer the best solution for continual movement. However, to challenge your ability to rapidly decelerate and stabilise, why not roll out and jump straight into a front support or push-up; for a more visually stunning effect (that is also physically challenging), roll out, plant the hands and kick up to handstand.

Exercise 10.4 Run to jumping on to an object

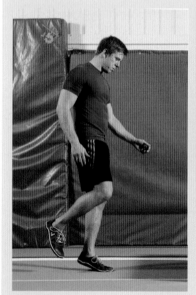 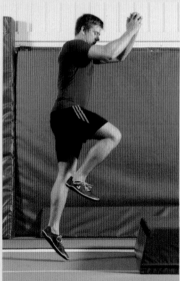 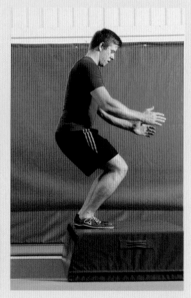

(a) Foot plant   (b) Pull through   (c) Land

The run to jump can be performed in several ways, depending on whether the objective is to jump on to or over an object (as seen in the images above), to clear a large distance, or to simply jump over several small obstacles while continuing to run (hurdling).

Basic movement

Running and jumping onto an object

- Run up to the object
- Plant one foot, bringing both arms back
- Swing the arms up and pull both feet through
- Land with both feet, and decelerate

Exercise 10.5 Hurdling over small objects

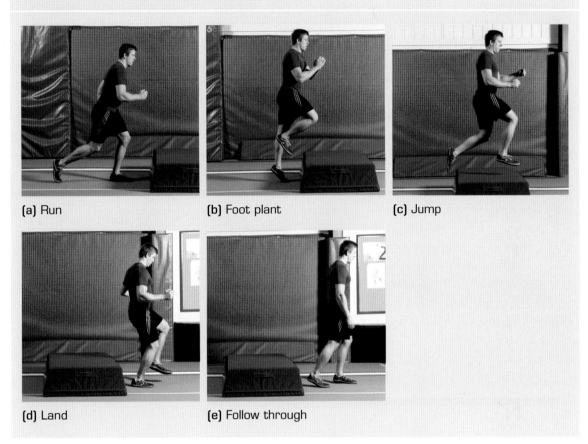

(a) Run   (b) Foot plant   (c) Jump

(d) Land   (e) Follow through

This sequence uses a single foot take off, as previously described.

- Run up to the object, lifting the lead leg to jump
- Look for a spot to land the lead foot and as you do, pull through the trail leg, land, and continue to run

Further explorations

- When jumping on to objects during a run, it's important to drill the foot plant, so you get a feel for where to plant the feet in front of the object. Taking off too close to an object runs the risk of hitting the object, and taking off too far away may result in missing the landing. The point at which you plant the feet should ideally be slightly in front of your centre of mass. Providing a tight hollow body shape is maintained, this will allow for a rapid translation of horizontal momentum into vertical momentum – resulting in more jump height. Taking off behind your centre of mass (i.e. leaning forwards) will start to rotate the body sooner and cause a loss of jump height.

- When jumping for distance (e.g. long jump), it may be useful to roll out of the landing (forward or shoulder roll). The exception to this is when jumping from one object to another, where a roll out is not possible (e.g. from one wall to another). These are known as precision jumps, and require a high degree of dynamic stability, spatial awareness and position sense.
- When hurdling over several small objects, it's important to maintain forward momentum and minimise any braking forces. As you jump, try flexing the trunk a little – just enough to keep the torso over the thigh. Furthermore, it's important to land the foot underneath the hips – at the point of foot strike, the trail leg should already be pulled through and ready to load. If foot strike occurs in front of the body and/or the trail leg remains behind the body, a significant braking force will occur causing an increased risk of injury to the lower extremity.

JUMPING AND VAULTING

Jumping and vaulting sequences demand higher levels of power, and it's important that this power requirement is built on a strong foundation of stability and strength. For this reason, ensure that you have mastered the basic supports, have a good level of whole body strength, and are competent in the basic jump progressions. Two sequences are explored here – the jump or drop down to roll, and the kong vault to roll.

Exercise 10.6 Drop down to roll

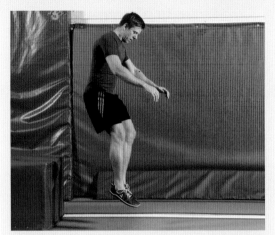

(a) Drop

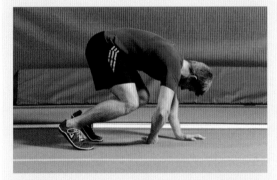

(b) Land

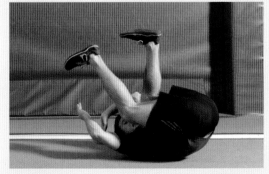

(c) Roll

The drop down to roll may feel awkward at first, but it's a useful skill to master, as it helps to drill efficient deceleration via a redistribution of force. When jumping from small heights, decelerating into a squat will often suffice; however, when landing from greater heights, a transition into a shoulder roll will help to distribute the impact force.

Basic movement

- As you jump down, aim to land evenly on two feet
- On landing, collapse (under control) into a squat as you lean forwards for the shoulder roll
- Reach the arm across the body and perform a shoulder roll back out to standing/running

Further explorations

- A common mistake when landing from greater heights is to drop vertically down. This will produce an immediate braking force, making it hard to redistribute this force quickly. Therefore, aim to jump out a little further, which will generate forward momentum on landing, and allow you to 'fall' into the roll. It's also important to land with your feet underneath your centre of mass to minimise braking forces, and potential risk of injury.
- Although the most obvious link out of this sequence is a return to upright standing or running, don't be afraid to explore other options. If you are jumping down from a relatively small height, try rolling out into a prone crawl pattern, or a jump to push-up/front support. From here, you can quickly link to any number of other bodyweight exercises and sequences.

Exercise 10.7 Kong vault to roll

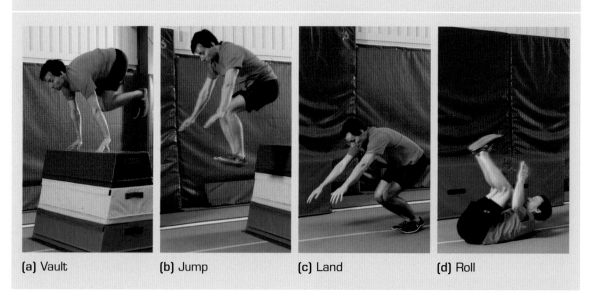

(a) Vault   **(b)** Jump   **(c)** Land   **(d)** Roll

This is another visually stunning sequence from the world of Parkour and free running, and is also a great bodyweight skill that is perfect for outdoor training programmes.

Basic movement

- Stand in front of a wall, railing or other suitable fixed obstacle, and position your hands ready for the vault
- Spot your landing place. When ready, push hard with the hands, lean forwards, and lift the hips up as you tuck the knees
- Release the hands and vault over the obstacle, aiming to land on two feet
- As you land, use the forward momentum to execute a shoulder roll

Further explorations

- To maintain forward momentum and efficiently clear the obstacle, the forward lean is crucial, and will help drive your centre of mass forwards. Initially, this can be a little daunting, as you may feel you will fall flat on your face. However, learning to quickly release the hands and pull the knees through will ensure a good landing that will allow an easy roll out.
- As confidence improves, you may wish to explore larger surfaces to traverse using the king vault, or even higher obstacles. In both cases, you will need to add a run up to the vault, as well as pay attention to the type of take off. For example, when vaulting over a longer obstacle, a single leg take off will help to maintain forward momentum, allowing you to plant the hands further down the obstacle. If you are looking to vault over a high obstacle, then after the run up, a two-footed punch will effectively translate forward momentum into vertical momentum. In both cases, don't forget to land and roll out with good technique.

QUADRUPEDAL

Crawling-based sequences are a growing trend within mainstream fitness training programmes, and much of this popularity has been influenced by their similarity to animal movements. From a conditioning perspective, there is no denying that moving about on all fours carries a high metabolic cost and provides a challenging training experience. When a variety of quadrupedal patterns are sequenced in fluid, imaginative ways, the result is a highly effective whole body-conditioning programme.

Exercise 10.8 Prone crawl to forward roll

Adding a roll to a crawl is a useful way to quickly cover a larger distance when crawling.

Basic movement

- Begin crawling in the usual way
- As you plant the lead hand, place the other hand next to it and push off the back leg into a forward roll

Further explorations

- Because you are entering the forward roll from a lower position, it's important to push off hard from the back leg. This will allow the hips (and centre of mass) to travel over the head with relative ease.
- Think about your next move after the roll. See how smoothly you can return to the crawl, or reach forwards into a front support. For power, roll out and jump into a burpee; and for flair, try rolling out and immediately jumping into a dive forward roll or cartwheel.

Exercise 10.8 Prone crawl to forward roll

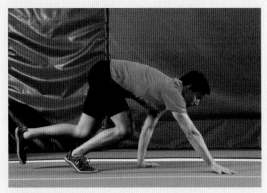

(a) Crawl

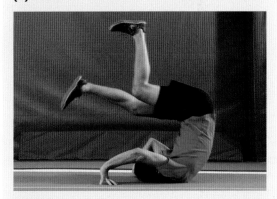

(b) Roll

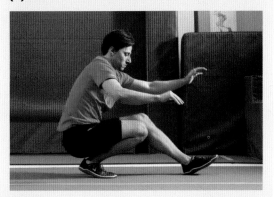

(c) Return to crawl

Exercise 10.9 Prone crawl to cartwheel

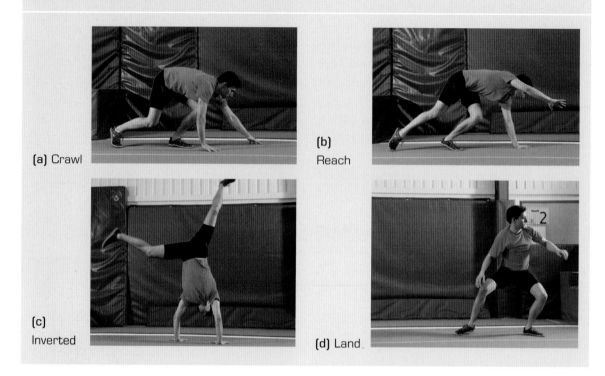

(a) Crawl

(b) Reach

(c) Inverted

(d) Land

In a similar way to the crawl to roll, the crawl to cartwheel requires maintainance forward momentum while simultaneously pulling the hips and legs over the head. Coordination of the hands and feet also provides an extra challenge.

Basic movement

- Begin the crawl in the usual way
- As you place the lead hand down, push off hard from the same side leg – this action will start to raise the hips up over the head
- Simultaneously reach the opposite hand across the body and plant it on the floor in front of the other, as you swing the back leg off the ground
- Push the ground away from you as you perform a cartwheel

Further explorations

- When you try this for the first time, it's worth slowing down the movement to learn the transition. Position yourself in the correct phase of the crawl, then practise jumping into the cartwheel. As you improve, you can build the crawl back in, until it becomes one continuous motion.
- Don't forget to explore your exit out of the cartwheel, which can either be into a side facing squat position, or facing the opposite direction to the crawl. Both exits have plenty of options to choose from, including a front/back sweep, sideways crawl/shuffle, prone crawl, dropping into a burpee, or a dive forward roll.

Exercise 10.10 Side shuffle to back sweep

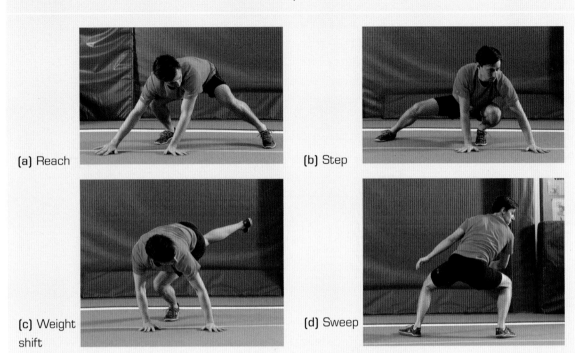

(a) Reach

(b) Step

(c) Weight shift

(d) Sweep

This is another capoeira-inspired sequence that works the whole body in all planes, and has plenty of style.

Basic movement
- On all fours, perform the side shuffle
- As the lead leg plants and you shift your bodyweight over, bend further over the leg and place your hands on the floor ready for the back sweep
- Perform the sweep, ending up facing the opposite direction

Further explorations
- This sequence can be drilled continuously to practise the movements on each side of the body. It can also be a useful transition move when deciding whether to drop to some ground-based movements or move to an upright position.

TUMBLING

Tumbling moves such as rolls and cartwheels generate large amounts of momentum that can be effectively transferred further horizontally, or even vertically. Whether these skills are performed for repetitions or integrated within longer movement sequences, the result is a highly challenging whole body workout that will reignite the senses. Two simple sequences will be discussed here that will motivate you to explore further.

Exercise 10.11 Forward roll to jump

This combination takes advantage of the transfer of forward momentum into vertical momentum. It also helps to train balance and spatial awareness.

Basic movement
- From standing, perform a forward roll
- As your feet plant, push hard into the ground and rapidly extend the arms up as you jump
- Keep a tight hollow shape as you jump up, and land in a balanced position ready for the next move

Further explorations
- For added power, try a dive forward roll to jump. Also, explore jump variations such as a roll to jump half-turn, full turn, tuck, or straddle jump. With a little bit of preparation, try a roll to jump over an object.

Exercise 10.11 Forward roll to jump

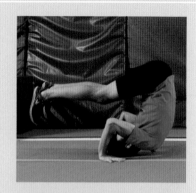

(a) Roll

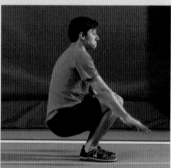

(b) Squat

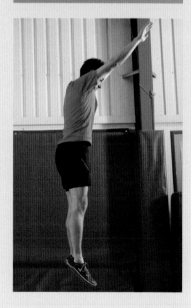

(c) Jump

Exercise 10.12 Roll to cartwheel

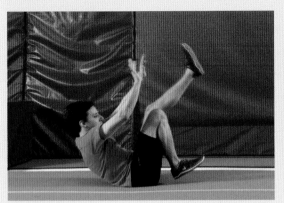

(a) Roll

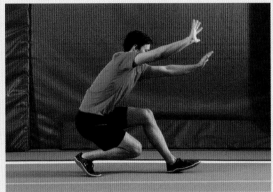

(b) Reach

In this combination, the momentum generated in the forward roll is effectively transferred to the cartwheel.

Basic movement
- Perform a roll (forward, dive or shoulder) aiming to land in a split stance
- Lunge out of the roll and push off the lead leg into a cartwheel to the same side

Further explorations
- Use the forward momentum of the roll to help you lean into the lunge at the start of the cartwheel.
- As you land out of the cartwheel, you can maintain momentum and flow of movement by adding a jump turn/step into a dive forward roll. Alternatively, performing a sweep, or a drop to front support/push-up will decelerate the movement, and bring you down to the floor in preparation for some ground-based movements.

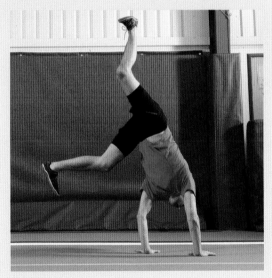

(c) Inverted

APPENDIX – SAMPLE WORKOUTS

WORKOUT TYPE	WHOLE BODY CONDITIONING			
WARM-UP	**10 minutes – neuromuscular activation, dynamic mobilisation, cardiorespiratory**			
MAIN SESSION				
Exercise	Sets	Reps	Duration/hold	NOTES
Deep squat	3	6–20		Drop as far as range of motion allows
Push-up	3	6–20		
Pull-up	3	6–20		
Lunges	2	6–20 each leg		Alternate legs or perform on one leg at a time
Inverted press	3	6–20		
Body row	3	6–20		Use a fixed bar, or suspension trainer
Front support	2	1	30 s	
Back support	2	1	30 s	
COOL DOWN	**5–10 minutes – dynamic movement, body rolling, functional flexibility**			
Progressions	Beginners: start with 6 reps per set, 30 s rest between sets			
	Intermediate: 12 reps per set, 30 s rest between sets			
	Advanced: 20 reps per set, 30 s rest between sets			
	Rest periods can be reduced instead of, or alongside, increases in reps.			

WORKOUT TYPE	LOWER-BODY CONDITIONING			
WARM-UP	**10 minutes – neuromuscular activation, dynamic mobilisation, cardiorespiratory**			
MAIN SESSION				
Exercise	Sets	Reps	Duration/hold	NOTES
Front scale	1	1	20 s	
Back scale	1	1	20 s	
Plyo bounces – 2 feet (180 bpm)	2	1	45 s	
Deep squat	3	6–20		
Single leg squat	2	6–20 each leg		
Side lunge	3	6–20 each leg		
Plyo bounces – 2 feet (180 bpm)	2	1	45 s	Use a metronome to maintain rhythm
Squat jump	2	6		
COOL DOWN	**5–10 minutes – dynamic movement, body rolling (lower body), functional flexibility**			
Progressions	Beginners: start with 6 reps per set, 30 s rest between sets			
	Intermediate: 12 reps per set, 30 s rest between sets			
	Advanced: 20 reps per set, 30 s rest between sets			
	Rest periods can be reduced instead of, or alongside, increases in reps.			

WORKOUT TYPE	UPPER-BODY CONDITIONING				
WARM-UP	**10 minutes – neuromuscular activation, dynamic mobilisation, cardiorespiratory**				
MAIN SESSION					
Exercise	Sets	Reps		Duration/hold	NOTES
Front support	2			20 s	
Back support	2			20 s	
Handstand	2			10 s	Against wall
Push-up	2	6–20			
Body row	2	6–20			Use a fixed bar, or suspension trainer
Inverted press	2	6–20			
Pull-up	2	6–20			
Dips	2	6–20			
Monster walk	2	15 steps each direction			
COOL DOWN	**5–10 minutes – dynamic movement, body rolling (upper-body), functional flexibility**				
Progressions	Beginners: start with 6 reps per set, 30 s rest between sets				
	Intermediate: 12 reps per set, 30 s rest between sets				
	Advanced: 20 reps per set, 30 s rest between sets				
	Rest periods can be reduced instead of, or alongside, increases in reps.				

WORKOUT TYPE	CORE CONDITIONING				
WARM-UP	**10 minutes – neuromuscular activation, dynamic mobilisation, cardiorespiratory**				
MAIN SESSION					
Exercise	Sets	Reps		Duration/hold	NOTES
Front support	2	1		20 s	
Side support	2	1		20 s	
Back support	2	1		20 s	
Super hero to hollow hold	1	8 each position		Hold each position for 2 s	Alternate continuously until you have completed 8 of each
Shoulder bridge	3	6–20			
Seated lift	1	6–20		1–2 s	
Hanging support	2	1		10 s	
Candlestick	2	6–20			
COOL DOWN	**5–10 minutes – dynamic movement, body rolling, functional flexibility**				
Progressions	Beginners: start with 6 reps per set, 30 s rest between sets				
	Intermediate: 12 reps per set, 30 s rest between sets				
	Advanced: 20 reps per set, 30 s rest between sets				
	Rest periods can be reduced instead of, or alongside, increases in reps.				

WORKOUT TYPE	CORE CONDITIONING			
WARM-UP	10 minutes – neuromuscular activation, dynamic mobilisation, cardiorespiratory			
MAIN SESSION				
Exercise	Sets	Reps	Duration/hold	NOTES
Front support	2	1	20 s	
Side support	2	1	20 s	
Back support	2	1	20 s	
Super hero to hollow hold	1	8 each position	Hold each position for 2 s	Alternate continuously until you have completed 8 of each
Shoulder bridge	3	6–20		
Seated lift	1	6–20	1–2 s	
Hanging support	2	1	10 s	
Candlestick	2	6–20		
COOL DOWN	5–10 minutes – dynamic movement, body rolling, functional flexibility			
Progressions	Beginners: start with 6 reps per set, 30 s rest between sets			
	Intermediate: 12 reps per set, 30 s rest between sets			
	Advanced: 20 reps per set, 30 s rest between sets			
	Rest periods can be reduced instead of, or alongside, increases in reps.			

METABOLIC CONDITIONING WORKOUTS

WORKOUT TYPE	WHOLE BODY REPETITION CIRCUIT			
WARM-UP	5–10 minutes – neuromuscular activation, dynamic mobilisation			
MAIN SESSION				
Exercise	Sets	Reps	Duration/hold	NOTES
Squat		8–20		Perform the exercises in the order shown as a circuit. Take no more than 20 s rest when moving from one to the other. At the end of the circuit take a 2 min rest. Repeat the circuit 3–5 times.
Push-up		8–20		
Lunge		8–20		
Pull-up		8–20		
Squat jump		8–20		
Inverted press		8–20		
Jumping jacks		8–20		
Body row		8–20		
Hollow body rock		8–20		
COOL DOWN	5–10 minutes – dynamic movement, body rolling, functional flexibility			
Progressions	Beginners: start with 8 reps per exercise			
	Intermediate: 15 reps per exercise			
	Advanced: 20 reps per exercise			
	Rest periods can be reduced instead of, or alongside, increases in reps.			

WORKOUT TYPE	WHOLE BODY TIMED CIRCUIT			
WARM-UP	**5–10 minutes – neuromuscular activation, dynamic mobilisation**			
MAIN SESSION				

Exercise	Sets	Reps	Duration/hold	NOTES
Squat		As many as possible	20–40 s	Perform the exercises in the order shown as a circuit. Take no more than 20 s rest when moving from one to the other. At the end of the circuit take a 2 min rest. Repeat the circuit 3–5 times.
Push-up			20–40 s	
Lunge			20–40 s	
Pull-up			20–40 s	
Squat jump			20–40 s	
Inverted press			20–40 s	
Jumping jacks			20–40 s	
Body row			20–40 s	
Hollow body rock			20–40 s	

COOL DOWN	**5–10 minutes – dynamic movement, body rolling, functional flexibility**
Progressions	Perform as many reps as possible in the time given. It's OK to rest during an exercise – just resume when you're ready.
	Beginners: start with 20 s per exercise
	Intermediate: 30 s per exercise
	Advanced: 40 s per exercise
	Rest periods can be reduced instead of, or alongside, increases in time.

WORKOUT TYPE	TABATA CIRCUIT – WHOLE BODY			
WARM-UP	**5–10 minutes – neuromuscular activation, dynamic mobilisation**			
MAIN SESSION				

Exercise	Sets	Reps	Duration/hold	NOTES
Squat		As many as possible	20 s	Perform the exercises in the order shown as a circuit. Take 10 s rest before moving on to the next. At the end of the circuit take a 2 min rest.
Kick through (alternate)			20 s	
Fast heel pulls			20 s	
Burpee			20 s	
Jumping jacks			20 s	
Push-ups			20 s	
Squat jumps			20 s	
Super hero rock			20 s	

COOL DOWN	**5–10 minutes – dynamic movement, body rolling, functional flexibility**
Progressions	As your fitness improves, perform more repetitions of the same circuit, or add other Tabata circuits.
	Don't be afraid to mix Tabata circuits with other forms of bodyweight training within a single workout.

WORKOUT TYPE	TABATA CIRCUIT – CORE			
WARM-UP	5–10 minutes – neuromuscular activation, dynamic mobilisation			
MAIN SESSION				
Exercise	Sets	Reps	Duration/hold	NOTES
Hollow body rock		As many as possible	20 s	Perform the exercises in the order shown as a circuit. Take 10 s rest before moving on to the next. At the end of the circuit take a 2 min rest.
Super hero rock			20 s	
Front support			20 s	
Back support			20 s	
Shoulder bridge			20 s	
Seat lift			20 s	
Candlestick			20 s	
Seated balance hold			20 s	
COOL DOWN	5–10 minutes – dynamic movement, body rolling, functional flexibility			
Progressions	As your fitness improves, perform more repetitions of the same circuit, or add other Tabata circuits.			
	Don't be afraid to mix Tabata circuits with other forms of bodyweight training within a single workout.			

BIOMOTOR SKILL-BASED WORKOUTS

WORKOUT TYPE	PLYOMETRIC TRAINING			
WARM-UP	10 minutes – neuromuscular activation, dynamic mobilisation			
MAIN SESSION				
Exercise	Sets	Reps	Duration/hold	NOTES
Jumping jacks		20–50		Perform these exercises as a circuit. Take 2 min rest, and repeat 3–5 times.
Explosive push-ups		6–12		
Tuck jumps		6–12		
Single leg bounces		30–60 each leg		
Burpees		6–12		
Squat jumps		8–10		
Kick through		6–12 each side		
Jump rope			2 minutes	
COOL DOWN	10 minutes – dynamic movement, body rolling, functional flexibility			
Progressions	Beginners should start at the lower end of the rep range, and increase reps as fitness improves.			

WORKOUT TYPE	ISOMETRIC STRENGTH/ENDURANCE TRAINING			
WARM-UP	**10 minutes – dynamic mobilisation, cardiorespiratory**			
MAIN SESSION				
Exercise	Sets	Reps	Duration/hold	NOTES
Front support	2		20–60 s	Perform these exercises as a circuit. Take 20 s rest between exercises and a 2 min rest at the end of the circuit. Repeat 3 times.
Side support	2		20–60 s	
Back support	2		20–60 s	
Hollow hold	2		20–60 s	
Shoulder bridge	2		20–60 s	
Seated balance	2		20–60 s	
Seat lift	2		20–60 s	
Crow	2		10–30 s	
Front scale	2		10–30 s	
Back scale	2		10–30 s	
COOL DOWN	**10 minutes – dynamic movement, body rolling, functional flexibility**			
Progressions	Beginners should start at the lower end of the duration/hold range, and increase time as endurance/strength improves.			

MOVEMENT SKILL-BASED WORKOUTS

WORKOUT TYPE	HANDSTAND PROGRESSIONS			
WARM-UP	**10 minutes – neuromuscular activation, dynamic mobilisation, cardiorespiratory**			
MAIN SESSION				
Exercise	Sets	Reps	Duration/hold	NOTES
Hollow body hold	5	1	20 s	Keep arms extended overhead; glutes and quads engaged.
Lunge with overhead reach	1	8 each side		Hold each lunge for a few seconds, keeping the arms overhead, abdominals engaged, and torso leaning forwards (in line with back leg).
Lunge, reach and plant	1	8 each side		Lunge (as above), and reach the hands forwards on the ground in front of you. As you reach, raise the back leg off the ground, so that when you plant the hands, you should still have the hollow shape.
Plant and kick	1	12 each side		With hands planted, push the support leg into the floor as you kick the back leg up. Maintain hollow shape throughout.
Kick up to split handstand	3	6 each side		Practise kicking up to handstand while keeping the legs split. This will allow you to get a feel for your balance point. Aim for a 5 s hold.
Kick to handstand	3	6 each side		Kick up to split handstand – hold for 5 s before slowly bringing the legs together.
COOL DOWN	**10 minutes – dynamic movement, body rolling, functional flexibility**			
Notes	The individual progressions described above are made up of each step towards kicking up to free standing handstand. It's important that you build up the required stability and strength using the building block exercises before working through the above drills.			

WORKOUT TYPE	FOUNDATION SKILLS TRAINING			
WARM-UP	**10 minutes – neuromuscular activation, dynamic mobilisation, cardiorespiratory**			
MAIN SESSION				
Exercise	Sets	Reps	Duration/hold	NOTES
L-sit	3–5	1	10 s	
Handstand	2	6	Up to 5 s	
Deep squat	3	10-15		
Muscle-up (rings)	3	3–6		
Burpee	3	3–6		
Candlestick	2	3–6		
Forward roll	2	3–6		
Prone crawl	3	1	20 s crawl	
Cartwheel	2	3–6		
COOL DOWN	**10 minutes – dynamic movement, body rolling, functional flexibility**			
Progressions	Increase repetitions as you improve.			
	Focus on maintaining the correct body shape/tension throughout each skill.			

PLAY/EXPLORATORY BASED WORKOUTS

WORKOUT THEME	EXPLORING LYING, SQUATTING AND FRONT SUPPORT
WARM-UP	**10 minutes – neuromuscular activation, dynamic mobilisation, cardiorespiratory**
MAIN SESSION	
Start position	**Explorations**
Lying supine	As you lie on your back, think about the different directions you can move in. Explore moving each arm and leg in all directions, noting how this motion affects the rest of your body. Notice how your head movement (lifting, rotating etc.) begins to set a direction for movement. Notice how reaching one arm to the opposite side or even overhead begins to rotate the torso. Moving the shoulder and head in the same direction will further drive this movement. Can you use all of these limbs to rotate on to your front? Can the legs also help to drive rotation in any way? How do you coordinate these body segments to create efficient rotation? Play around with these rotational movements for a while, looking for an efficient way to roll on to your front. Now begin to explore flexion. How can you efficiently move into a seated position? What sort of shapes do you have to form? Is there a way to use the arms or legs to help you sit up. Explore making a hollow shape with the torso and rocking back and forth. Does this help in any way towards sitting upright? Tuck your knees in and rock back and forth along your back. Can you generate enough momentum to rock into a seated position? As you move into the prone lying or seated positions, begin a new process of exploration. Where can you go from here? Each time you discover a new position, reverse the flow back to the start position. Notice whether the flow becomes blocked, and look for ways to unblock the movement so it becomes fluid.

Deep squat	Position yourself comfortably in a deep squat, and begin to think about where you can go from here.
	Begin with some arm movements. Try reaching each arm up – notice the torso rotation it produces. What happens to the rotation potential if you push the opposite arm into the floor? As you reach up with one arm, see how far you can reach backwards. What do your hips have to do in order to reach further back? Try it on the other side.
	Now reach your hands forwards and to the sides. Where does this begin to take you?
	Now explore some hip movements. Drive one hip and knee forwards. What does your opposite foot have to do to allow this to happen? As you drive the hip and knee forward, where does your body want to go? Can you drive the opposite hip/knee forward from here? See if you can link several of these movements together.
	In the deep squat position, try sliding one leg out to the side. Where does your weight shift when you do this? Try sliding/stepping one leg forwards. Is there a way to efficiently transfer your bodyweight on to this leg? How can your torso help out with this movement?
	Play around with some other linking movements from the deep squat. Try placing your hands on the floor behind you. Where can you go from here? Place your hands on the floor in front of you and transfer some weight on to them so that you are in a prone crawl position. Where can you go from here? Finally, reach your hands to the side. Where can you go from here? As you link new movements, don't forget to reverse the sequence back to the start position.
Front support	Assume a front support position, and think about potential directions for movement. What happens when you lift one arm towards the ceiling? Which way does your body want to go? Continue moving in that direction, noticing what you have to do to maintain balance and flow.
	Try reaching one arm forwards. Is this enough to drive the body forwards? What else has to move if you want to go forwards?
	From front support, allow the arms and legs to bend a little. How does this feel? Is this a better position from which to move? Explore ways to move forwards/backwards/sideways from here.
	Is there a way to move efficiently between the front support, deep squat and supine lying? Are any transitional movements required to maintain the flow? Can you move forwards through this sequence as well as backwards?
COOL DOWN	**5–10 minutes – dynamic movement, body rolling, functional flexibility**

REFERENCES AND FURTHER READING

REFERENCES

Caterisano A, Moss RF, Pellinger TK, Woodruff K, Lewis VC, Booth W, Khadra T (2002). The effect of back squat depth on the EMG activity of 4 superficial hip and thigh muscles. *Journal of Strength and Conditioning Research* 16(3): 428–32

Chandler T, Wilson G, Stone M (1989). The effect of the squat exercise on knee stability. *Medicine & Science in Sports & Exercise* 21(3): 299-303

Clark MA and Lucett SC (2011). *NASM's Essentials of Corrective Exercise Training*. 1st ed. Philadelphia: Wolters Kluwer Health/Lippincott Williams & Wilkins

Klein K (1961). The deep squat exercise as utilised in weight training for athletes and its effects on the ligaments of the knee. *Journal of the Association for Physical and Mental Rehabilitation* 15(1): 6–11

Li G, Rudy TW, Sakane M, Kanamori A, Ma CB, Woo SL (1999). The importance of quadriceps and hamstring muscle loading on knee kinematics and in-situ forces in the ACL. *Journal of Biomechanics* 32(4): 395–400

Li G, Zayontz S, Most E, DeFrate LE, Suggs JF, Rubash HE (2004). In situ forces of the anterior and posterior cruciate ligaments in high knee flexion: an in vitro investigation. *Journal of Orthopaedic Research* 22(2): 293–7

Markolf KL, Slauterbeck JL, Armstrong KL, Shapiro MM, Finerman GA (1996). Effects of combined knee loadings on posterior cruciate ligament force generation. *Journal of Orthopaedic Research* 14 (4): 633–8

Meyers E (1971). Effect of selected exercise variables on ligament stability and flexibility of the knee. *Research Quarterly* 42(4): 411–422

Panariello R, Backus S, Parker J (1994). The effect of the squat exercise on anterior-posterior knee translation in professional football players. *American Journal of Sports Medicine* 22(6): 768-773

Sakane M, Fox RJ, Woo SL, Livesay GA, Li G, Fu FH (1997). In situ forces in the anterior cruciate ligament and its bundles in response to anterior tibial loads. *Journal of Orthopaedic Research* 15 (2): 285–93

Steiner M, Grana W, Chilag K, Schelberg-Karnes E (1986). The effect of exercise on anterior-posterior knee laxity. *American Journal of Sports Medicine* 14(1): 24–29

Tabata I, Nishimura K, Kouzaki M, Hirai Y, Ogita F, Miyachi M, Yamamoto K (1996). Effects of moderate-intensity endurance and high-intensity intermittent training on anaerobic capacity and VO_2max. *Medicine & Science in Sports Exercise* 28(10): 1327–30

Taunton JE, Ryan MB, Clement DB, McKenzie DC, Lloyd-Smith DR, Zumbo BD (2003). A prospective study of running injuries: the Vancouver Sun Run 'In Training' clinics. *British Journal of Sports Medicine* 37: 239–44

van Gent RM, Siem D, van Middlekoop M, van Os A.G, Bierma-Zeinstra AMA, Koes BW (2007). Incidence and determinants of lower extremity running injuries in long distance runners: a systematic review. *British Journal of Sports Medicine* 41: 469–80

van Mechelen W (1992). Running injuries. A review of the epidemiological literature. *Sports Medicine* 14: 320–335

FURTHER READING

Clark MA and Lucett SC (2011). *NASM's Essentials of Corrective Exercise Training*, 1st ed. Philadelphia: Wolters Kluwer Health/Lippincott Williams & Wilkins

Feldenkrais M (2003). *The Potent Self: A Study of Spontaneity and Compulsion*, New Ed. North Atlantic Books

Feldenkrais M (2005). *Body and Mature Behaviour: A Study of Anxiety, Sex, Gravitation and Learning*, Revised Ed. North Atlantic Books

Hébert G (1912). *L'éducation physique ou l'entrainement complet par la méthode naturelle*, Librairie Vuibert

Low S (2011). *Overcoming Gravity: A systematic approach to gymnastic and bodyweight strength*, CreateSpace Independent Publishing Platform

Patel K (2008). *The Complete Guide to Postural Training*, A&C Black

Saxby L (2012). *Proprioception: Making Sense of Barefoot Running*, Vivobarefoot.com

Siff MC (2003). *Supertraining*, 6th ed. Denver: Supertraining Institute

Zake Y and Golden S (1997). *Body Rolling: An experiential approach to complete muscle release*, Vermont: Healing Arts Press

GLOSSARY

Acute exercise variables – the factors that can be manipulated to affect the outcome of any exercise, i.e. reps, sets, load, rest period etc.

Adaptive capacity – the capacity of a system to adapt if the environment where the system exists is changing

Anaerobic capacity – the total amount of energy obtainable from the anaerobic energy systems

Angle of pull – angle between the muscle insertion and the bone on which it pulls

Appendicular skeleton – the part of the skeleton that includes the shoulder girdle, pelvic girdle, and the upper and lower limbs

Aston Patterning – a blend of movement education, structural bodywork, and fitness to facilitate rehabilitation, improve athletic performance and prevent injury, developed by dancer Judith Aston

Axial skeleton – the part of the skeleton that includes the skull, spinal column, sternum and ribs

Balance – an even distribution of weight enabling a body to remain upright and stable

Biomechanics – the study of the mechanical laws relating to the movement or structure of living organisms

Biomotor skills – the specific skills or abilities that affect fitness, e.g. strength, power, speed, endurance, flexibility etc.

Body rolling – a set of techniques that involve self-myofascial release used to inhibit overactive muscles and improve soft tissue extensibility

Body tension – a term used in gymnastics that refers to a body being held tight

Brachiation – to move by swinging with the arms from one hold to another

Cadence – the measure or beat of movement

Capoeira – an Afro-Brazilian art form that combines elements of martial arts, music and dance

Cardiorespiratory system – a body system composed of the cardiovascular system and the respiratory system, including the heart, lungs and blood vessels

Centre of mass – unique point at the centre of a body around which mass is balanced

Comfort zone – a place or situation where one feels safe or at ease and without stress

Contralateral – belonging to or occurring on the opposite side of the body

Cool down – a period following strenuous physical activity in which milder exercise is performed to allow the body to gradually return to normal

Coordination – the ability to repeatedly execute a sequence of movements smoothly and accurately

Cortisol – a hormone made in the adrenal glands and released in response to stress

CrossFit – a strength and conditioning brand and exercise programme that combines elements of weight lifting, sprinting and gymnastics in a high intensity, functional manner

Dorsiflexion – a movement where the top of the foot is moved towards the tibia

Efficiency – a level of performance that describes a process of completing a task with the highest economy of effort

Endurance – the ability to exert (sub maximal) force over an extended period of time

Evolution – the gradual change in the characteristics of a population over successive generations

Exit strategy – an exercise or movement that allows safe transition out of another movement

Extensibility – capable of being stretched

Extension – a physical position that increases the angle between the bones of the limb at a joint

Fascia – a sheet or band of fibrous connective tissue enveloping, separating, or binding together muscles, organs and other soft tissues

Feldenkrais Method – a somatic educational system designed by Moshé Feldenkrais, to reduce pain or limitations in movement and to improve physical function

Flexibility – the range of motion in a joint or group of joints

Flexion – a physical position that decreases the angle between the bones of the limb at a joint

Ginastica Natural – a complete bodyweight training method developed by Alvaro Romano, that develops physical qualities such as strength, power, endurance, mobility, balance and coordination using ancient, modern and natural techniques

Gravity – the force that attracts a body toward the centre of the earth, or toward any other physical body having mass

Greasing the groove – a technique pioneered by renowned strength and conditioning coach, Pavel Tsatsouline, that focuses on combining specificity of movement with repetition

Gross motor skills – the abilities acquired during early childhood as part of a child's motor development

Ground reaction force – any force exerted by the ground on a body in contact with it

Growth hormone – a hormone that stimulates cellular growth

Gymnastics – physical exercises designed to develop and display strength, balance and control

Hanna Somatics – a form of neuromuscular movement re-education that addresses chronic patterns of muscular contraction

Heuristic – allowing a person to discover or learn something for themselves

High intensity intermittent/interval training (HIIT) – a form of training that involves cycles of high intensity bursts and low to moderate intensity recovery

Insulin – a hormone produced in the pancreas that regulates the amount of glucose in the blood

Intensity – the amount of effort or work that must be invested in a specific exercise or workout

Ipsilateral – belonging to or occurring on the same side of the body

Isometric – a muscle action in which the joint angle and muscle length do not change during contraction

Kipping – a manoeuvre that combines a hip drive and kick to generate momentum during a pull-up

Lactic acid – an organic acid produced in muscle tissues during strenuous activity

Locomotion – movement, or the ability to move from one place to another

Manipulative skill – a skilful movement done to or with objects, e.g. pushing, pulling, throwing etc.

Maximal voluntary contraction – the greatest amount of tension a muscle can generate

Metabolic conditioning – any type of conditioning that increases the storage and delivery of energy for any activity and improves the efficiency of the different metabolic pathways

Midline stability – relating to stability of the entire spine

Mobilisation – movement of a joint, either passively or actively (dynamic)

Momentum – force of movement, or 'mass in motion', equal to mass multiplied by velocity

Motor development – the step by step development of a child's gross and fine motor skills, including movement control, flexibility, dexterity, and exploration

Musculoskeletal system – the system of muscles, tendons, ligaments, bones, joints and associated tissues that move the body and maintain its form

Neuromuscular activation – the process by which the nervous system produces muscular force through recruitment and rate coding of motor units

Neuromuscular system – the combination of the nervous system and the muscles, working together to allow movement

Over-reaching – an accumulation of training stress that results in a short-term decrease in functional capacity

Overtraining – an accumulation of training stress that results in a long-term decrease in capacity

Paraspinal – adjacent to the spinal column

Parkour – a physical discipline of training that involves moving quickly and efficiently over environmental obstacles

Plantarflexion – a movement which increases the angle between the front part of the foot and the tibia

Play – physical or mental activity that is undertaken purely for enjoyment or amusement and has no other objective

Plyometrics – a form of exercise involving repeated rapid stretching and contracting of muscles, commonly used to increase power

Posture – the configuration and organisation of body segments at any given time

Power – the ability to exert a maximal force in as short a time as possible

Prime mover muscle – a muscle that acts directly to produce a desired movement

Prone – in a position face downward

Proprioception – the ability to sense the position, location, movement and orientation of the body and its parts

Propulsion – the action of pushing or driving forward

Quadrupedal locomotion – a terrestrial movement pattern using four limbs or legs

Range of motion (ROM) – the distance and direction a joint can move between the flexed position and the extended position

Repetitions – the number of times an exercise is performed

Rotation – the process of turning around an axis; in exercise, this may relate to isolated joint motion, or to the body as a whole unit

Sacrum – a triangular bone in the lower back located between the two innominate bones of the pelvis

Scalable – able to be changed in size to accommodate progression

Sequential – performed or used in sequence

Sets – the number of times an exercise or movement is repeated for a given number of repetitions

Skill – the ability and capacity (acquired through deliberate and systematic effort) to carry out complex activities or functions smoothly and adaptively.
Read more: http://www.businessdictionary.com/definition/skill.html#ixzz2gHqCf6V1

Soft tissue – tissues that connect, support, or surround other structures and organs of the body, including tendons, ligaments, fascia, skin, fibrous tissues, fat, muscles, nerves and blood vessels

Stability – resistance to change of position; in the context of motor development, one of three gross motor skills developed in early life

Static stretching – techniques used to stretch muscles while the body is at rest

Strength – the ability to exert force using muscular contraction

Supine – in a position face upward

Tabata training – a training protocol developed by Professor Izumi Tabata that uses 20 seconds of ultra-intense exercise followed by 10 seconds of rest, repeated continuously for 4 minutes (8 cycles)

Testosterone – a steroid hormone that stimulates development of male secondary sexual characteristics

Thoracic spine – the middle segment of the vertebral column between the cervical and lumbar spine, consisting of 12 vertebrae

Transitional – relating to the process of changing from one position to another

Unilateral – relating to, or affecting only one side of the body

Warm-up – a set of exercises or activities that consist of a gradual increase in intensity that help to prepare the body for the tasks ahead

INDEX